A Guide to Flexible Dieting

How Being Less Strict with Your Diet Can Make it Work Better

Lyle McDonald

This book is not intended for the treatment or prevention of disease, nor as a substitute for medical treatment, nor as an alternative to medical advice. It is a review of scientific evidence presented for information purposes only. Use of the guidelines herein is at the sole choice and risk of the reader.

Copyright: © 2005 by Lyle McDonald. All rights reserved.

This book or any part thereof, may not be reproduced or recorded in any form without permission in writing from the publisher, except for brief quotations embodied in critical articles or reviews.

For information contact:
Lyle McDonald Publishing
PO Box 1713
Salt Lake City, Ut 84110
Email: lylemcd@comcast.net

Cover and interior book design by Jazz Kalsi
Email: jkalsi@gmail.com

ISBN: 978-0-9671456-5-5

FIRST EDITION
FIRST PRINTING

Acknowledgments

My main acknowledgments go out to my innumerable guinea pigs and test subjects who have helped me develop some of my ideas, especially regarding structured refeeds.

Beyond that, I'm only going to acknowledge my own completion of 2 books at the same time. Trust me, I deserve it.

Table of Contents

Introduction

This is not your father's diet book 1

A brief tangent: Weight vs. Fat loss 5

Why Diets Fail Part 1 9

Why Diets Fail Part 2 15

How dieters fail diets 17

How diets fail dieters 21

Introduction to Flexible Dieting 27

Determining your body fat percentage 33

Free meals 37

Structured refeeds Part 1 41

Structured Refeeds Part 2 47

The Full Diet Break 57

Eating at Maintenance 67

Ending the Diet Approach 1 73

Eating at Maintenance 85

Moving Back Into Dieting 97

Appendix 1: BMI and Body fat estimation charts 105

Introduction

See if this sounds familiar: you've just started a new diet, certain that it's going to be different this time around and that it's going to work. You're cranking along, adjust to the new eating (and exercise) patterns and everything is going just fine. For a while.

Then the problem hits. Maybe it's something small, a slight deviation or dalliance. There's a bag of cookies and you have one or you're at the mini mart and just can't resist a little something that's not on your diet. Or maybe it's something a little bit bigger, a party or special event comes up and you know you won't be able to stick with your diet. Or, at the very extreme, maybe a vacation comes up, a few days out of town or even something longer, a week or two. What do you do?

Now, if you're in the majority, here's what happens: You eat the cookie and figure that you've blown your diet and might as well eat the entire bag. Clearly you were weak willed and pathetic for having that cookie, the guilt sets in and you might as well just start eating and eating and eating.

Or since the special event is going to blow your diet, you might as well eat as much as you can and give up, right? The diet is obviously blown by that single event so might as well chuck it all in the garbage. Vacations can be the ultimate horror, it's not as if you're going to go somewhere special for 3 days (or longer) and stay on your diet, right? Might as well throw it all out now and just eat like you want, gain back all the weight and then some.

What if I told you that none of the above had to happen? What if I told you that expecting to be perfect on your diet was absolutely setting you up for failure, that being more flexible about your eating habits would make them work better? What if I told you that studies have shown that people who are flexible dieters (as opposed to rigid dieters) tend to weigh less, show better adherence to their diet in the long run and have less binge eating episodes?

What if I told you that deliberately fitting in 'free' (or cheat or reward) meals into your diet every week would make it work better in the long run, that deliberately overeating for 5-24 hours can sometimes be a necessary part of a diet (especially for active individuals), that taking 1-2 weeks off of your diet to eat normally may actually make it easier to stick with in the long run in addition to making it work better.

I can actually predict that your response is one of the following. Some may think I'm making the same set of empty promises that every other book out there makes. But I have the data and real-world experience to back up my claims. Or, maybe the idea of making your diet less strict and miserable is something you actively resist. I've run into this with many dieters; they seem to equate suffering and misery with success and would rather doom themselves to failure by following the same pattern that they've always followed rather than consider an alternate approach. Finally, maybe what little I wrote above makes intuitive sense to you and you want to find out more.

Regardless of your reaction to what I've written, I already have your money so you might as well read on.

I should probably warn you that this isn't a typical diet book. You won't find a lot of rah-rah or motivational types of writing, there are no food lists and no recipes. There are thousands of other books out there which fit that bill if that's what you want but this isn't it.

This is not your father's diet book

I want to make it very clear that the booklet you're holding in your hand is not a diet book by any sort of conventional definition. You won't find food lists or recipes in most of my books (I made a slight concession in the Rapid Fat Loss Handbook) and certainly not in this one.

Rather, this book is more about some of the psychological and behavioral aspects of dieting. I'll introduce you to the concepts of flexible versus rigid dieting, free meals, structured refeeds and even full, two-week diet breaks. All of these are strategies to help you, in the long run, stay on your diet and maintaining the weight that you worked so hard to lose. And although I will make a few comments about dieting in general, within the context of this booklet I'm not going to tell you to follow this, that or the other diet.

Losing weight: The bottom line

Regardless of the nonsense you read in most diet books, losing weight is not fundamentally difficult. In my honest opinion, the last 30 years of research has told us all we really need to know about the topic. My grandmother knew how to lose weight before that but everybody knows that grandmothers know everything.

The bottom (and rather simple) line is that you have to adjust your food intake (or activity levels) so that you're burning more calories than you take in. Over time, this causes you to lose weight (I'll be making a distinction between weight and fat loss in the next chapter). That's really it and I've joked that my job is to turn the idea "Eat less, exercise, and repeat forever" into a 300 page book. One of these days I'll write/finish my magnum opus but for right now, this is what you get.

Even the books that tell you that you don't have to count calories still ultimately trick you into eating less, by adjusting what you can eat (and sometimes when you can eat it). Low-carbohydrate, low-fat, the Zone, you name a diet and they are making you eat less food in the long run. There's simply no way to escape that, no matter what magic they promise. Other weight loss approaches take the exercise route, get you burning more calories through activity under the assumption that you won't just eat more to compensate (which tends to be a rather bad assumption most of the time). There's really nothing magical to weight loss no matter what you want to believe.

Quite in fact, no weight loss study ever has found people who don't lose some amount of weight. They all do even though weight loss varies quite a bit between individuals (for a variety of reasons). All of the people you know (or you yourself) who have dieted have lost weight, too. You can't deny that. Eat less or exercise more and you will lose some amount of weight. How much depends on several factors depending on the severity of the diet, how long you stay on it, gender, genetics and a host of other stuff. But, fundamentally, losing weight is not difficult. Eat less, exercise (or both), repeat forever. That's the bottom line and the sooner you accept that the closer you'll be too reaching your goal.

So what's the problem?

You've probably heard the statistic that something like 95% of people regain all of the weight that they've lost within a few years. While this exact number may or may not be correct, the general concept is: most people who lose weight (through any method) will gain it all back within some period of time (months to a few years). Sometimes they gain back more weight than they started with and end up even fatter. Now, a number of groups use this statistic to claim that 'Diets don't make you lose weight' but that's completely inaccurate. Any diet that alters your energy intake (food) to expenditure (activity) will cause you to lose weight.

It's simply that most people don't maintain that weight loss in the long run. They lose it, but then they gain it all back (or more). Or at least gain back some proportion of it back. This is an important distinction that must be made: it is not that diets don't cause weight loss, they all do. Most dieters simply regain all the weight that they lose back.

As I stated above, research has been looking at different diets, different nutrients to see what diet is 'best' for losing weight. Well, there is no absolute best, it depends on the person. Activity levels, food preferences, gender, genetics all seem to affect which diet is 'best' for a given person (although there are some generalities that all diets must meet that I'll address later). About the best summary I've seen is that, if there is an optimal diet for the treatment of obesity, it should contain plenty of lean protein, lots of high fiber vegetables and fruits, moderate amounts of refined starches and moderate amounts of fat. Yippee, 30 years and millions of dollars of research to conclude what my grandmother knew all along.

In any event, asking which diet is best for weight loss is the wrong question to be asking in the first place as far as I'm concerned. At this point in the game, we know how to make people lose weight: you get them to eat less, get them to move more, and get them to repeat that forever. Yes, certainly research is showing that some approaches work better than others (though no single approach can be right for everybody in my opinion) but that's all water under the bridge, we know most of what we need to know about causing weight loss to occur.

So the problem is not weight loss; rather, the problem is with maintenance of weight loss. Researchers have to figure out how to get people to keep the weight/fat off that they lost in the long term. The issue has more to do with long-term adherence to diet and activity changes, not so much what those changes should be.

To me, that's the far more interesting (and complicated) question: why are people so poor at maintaining weight loss? More generally, why do most people fail at changing most behaviors. That is, a severe failure rate is not isolated to weight loss, the simple fact is that most people will fail to change any of their long-standing behavior patterns. Whether it's drinking, drug use, smoking, eating or their exercise patterns, most people will revert back to their old patterns fairly quickly.

In my opinion, the diet people (or the alcohol or drug people) need to get the psychology/behavioral people into the game, figure out why people are just so damn resistant to long-term behavior change. Figure that out and you've solved most of the problems. Since I don't think that answer is coming any time soon, I can only present the data I currently have to work with in this regards.

So what's the solution?

I'd either be delusional or the ultimate egotist (some of my critics would say I'm both) to think I had the complete solution to the problems that face dieters. If I had some nifty magic trick (which is what all diet books claim to have) for quick, easy weight loss or just told you that I did, I'd be a much richer man. I don't and I won't pretend that I do. There are no guarantees and nothing I am going to present in this booklet should be construed or misconstrued as such.

However, there are certain types of behaviors that are associated with greater success rates in terms of dieting or exercise programs or what have you. Don't misunderstand me, you'll still have to work and dieting is no fun no matter how you cut it. In the long-term, you still have to adjust your overall food intake, you'll probably have to adjust your activity levels. That doesn't change and nothing I can say or do changes that.

What I mainly want to talk about is ways to make the reality of long-term dieting, the 'repeat forever' part a little easier to cope with psychologically. But I'm getting ahead of myself, this is just an introductory chapter. The good stuff starts next.

4

A brief tangent: Weight vs. Fat loss

Although this trend is changing recently, most diet books tend to only talk about weight loss and I suspect that most dieters only think in terms of weight loss. In this chapter, I want to make a distinction between weight loss and fat loss before moving on to the meat of this particular booklet.

If you have my Rapid Fat Loss Handbook, you'll recognize this as being the exact same text reused (why should I bother rewriting the same information) and you can skip to the next chapter. If you aren't aware of the distinction between body weight and body fat (and weight loss versus fat loss), please keep reading.

Weight versus fat loss: They are not the same thing

Every tissue in your body (including muscle, body fat, your heart, liver, spleen, kidneys, bones, water, minerals etc.) weighs a given amount. We could (conceivably anyhow) take each of them out of your body, plop them on a scale and find out how much they weigh. Your total body weight is comprised of the weight of every one of those tissues. But only some portion of the total weight is fat.

For this reason, researchers and techie types frequently divide the body into two (or more) components including fat mass (the sum total of the body fat you have on your body) and lean body mass (everything else). While there are different 'types' of body fat (a topic to be discussed in an upcoming book project), this is more detail than we need.

Let's say that we could magically determine the weight of only your fat cells. Of course, we know your total weight by throwing you on a scale. By dividing the total amount of fat into the total body weight, you can determine a body fat percentage which represents the percentage of your total weight is fat.

Lean athletes might only have 5-10% body fat, meaning that only 5-10% of their total weight is fat. So a 200 pound athlete with 10% body fat is carrying 20 lbs. (200 * 0.10 = 20) of body fat. The remaining 180 pounds (200 total pounds - 20 pounds of fat weight = 180 lbs.) is muscle, organs, bones, water, etc. Researchers call the remaining 180 pounds lean body mass or LBM. I'll be using LBM a lot so make sure and remember what it means: LBM is lean body mass, the amount of your body that is not fat.

In cases of extreme obesity, a body fat percentage of 40-50% or higher is not unheard of. Meaning that nearly one-half of that person's total weight is fat. A 400 pound person with 50% body fat is carrying 200 lbs. of body fat. The other 200 pounds is muscle, organs, bones, etc. Again, 200 pounds of LBM along with 200 pounds of fat.

Most people fall somewhere between these two extremes. An average male may carry from 18-23% body fat and an average female somewhere between 25-30% body fat. So a male at 180 lbs. and 20% body fat is carrying 36 pounds of fat and the rest of his weight (144 lbs.) is LBM. A 150 pound female at 30% body fat has 50 pounds of body fat and 100 pounds of LBM.

Healthy levels of body fat are somewhat up to debate but most 'authorities' recommend 11-18% as being optimally healthy for males and 18-25% as being optimal for females. And, yes, this means that being too lean can have its own set of health problems as well but being too lean is generally not the problem for the average diet book reader (I'm not trying to be mean here, just making a statement of fact).

I want to point out that even if you never achieve 'healthy' body fat levels, even a small fat loss (10% of your current weight) can vastly improve health. So if you currently weigh 250 and lose even 25 lbs. and keep it off long-term, you will be healthier even if you are still above 'optimal' body fat percentage levels.

Why is this important?

So let's say you start a diet, reducing some part of your daily food intake. Maybe you start exercising, too. After some time period, you get on the scale and it says you've lost 10 lbs.. That's 10 lbs. of weight. But how much of it is fat? Frankly, you have no way of knowing with just the scale (unless it's one of those Tanita body fat scales, which attempt to estimate body fat percentage but don't work very well in my opinion). You could have lost fat or muscle or just dropped a lot of water. Even a big bowel movement can cause a weight loss of a pound or two (or more, depending). A colonic that clears out your entire lower intestinal tract may cause a significant weight loss. The scale can't tell you what you've lost, it can only tell you how much you have lost.

When you're worrying about long-term changes, the real goal is fat loss (some LBM loss is occasionally acceptable but that's more detail than I want to get into here). That is, cycling water weight on and off of your body (as frequently happens with certain dieting approaches) isn't really moving you towards any real goal even if makes you think you are. Don't get me wrong, it may be beneficial in the short-term (I mentioned a few of those situations in The Rapid Fat Loss Handbook) but it doesn't represent true fat loss.

In my last booklet, I brought up this issue since the diet I was describing tends to cause both rapid fat and weight losses (from water weight loss) and I wanted readers to be clear of the distinction. I mainly bring this issue up in this booklet because I'm going to have you get a rough estimate of your body fat percentage later in this book. That estimate will be used to determine how to use the varying flexible dieting strategies I'm going to describe. For that reason, a basic understanding of body fat percentage is necessary.

The real take home message of this chapter is this: your body can be divided up into two major components, lean body mass (or LBM) and fat mass. The total amount of fat you are carrying divided by your total body weight gives us your body fat percentage. I could have just written that short paragraph and skipped everything else but I have to justify the cost of this booklet somehow.

8

Why Diets Fail Part 1
Body weight Regulation

I mentioned in Chapter 1 the rather dismal success rates for weight loss (and most types of behavior change). Again, the typically claimed statistic for dieters is that 95% will regain all of the weight that they lost within a few years. The reasons why are the topic this and the next few chapters.

Now, one of the longer standing debates, with a lot of flip-flopping over the years is whether diets are failing for biological or psychological reasons. Now, first off let me say that the distinction is a false one and you can't ever separate the two: biology affects psychology and psychology affects biology.

However, for the purpose of this discussion and this booklet, I'm going to make that very separation. Just realize that I'm only making it for convenience. At the end of the day, both biological and psychological factors are interacting and solving (or even trying to solve) the problems associated with long-term weight maintenance mean dealing with both.

In this chapter, I want to deal with the biology of dieting and body weight regulation (this will make more sense in a second), in the next chapter, I'm going to deal with some of the more psychological/behavioral factors that tend to make long-term weight loss an issue. I should note that if you've read either of my other two booklets (Bromocriptine or The Ultimate Diet 2.0), you can probably skip most of this, there's nothing much new here. If not, please read this chapter first.

What is regulation?

To understand what I'm talking about when I refer to body weight regulation, I should probably define what it means for a system to be regulated in the first place. When a system is regulated, that means that it attempts (through whatever means) to maintain itself around some predetermined level. The example I've used over the years is of the thermostat in your house so that's what I'm going to use here.

So let's say that you set the thermostat to some temperature, let's choose 70 degrees. Now, the thermostat has a thermometer in it which is keeping track of the temperature. If the temperature goes much below 70 degrees, the heat turns on; if it goes much above 70 degrees, the air conditioner comes on. The end result is that the temperature in your house will stay, within some range, around the temperature you have set the thermostat to. That's a regulated system.

You can probably think of other regulated systems, an easy example might be the cruise control in your car. You set it to a certain speed and the car has a measurement device that changes how much gas is going to the engine depending on your speed: when the car slows down, more gas is given so that you speed up; when you start going too fast, less gas is given (or the brake is applied).

Of course, in both systems, the change in output (temperature or speed) changes the input, which is how the system stays regulated: it's just a giant loop. So the temperature drops, the thermostat senses it, the heat comes on, which increases the temperature, which the thermostat senses, turning the heat off. Schematically, the system looks like the following.

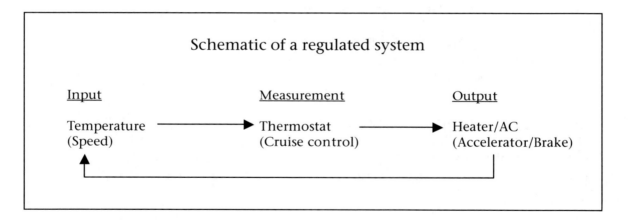

Body weight regulation

Now, many, if not most systems in the human body are regulated. Consider body temperature where the body strives to maintain a rather normal level (98.6 Fahrenheit in the US, I have no idea what that is in Celsius). If you are put somewhere cold, your body will make you shiver, as well as cutting off blood flow to your extremities (this is why fingers and toes get so cold) to try and keep your body heat up. Go into the heat or exercise and your body sweats and increases blood flow to the extremities to try and get rid of the excess heat so that you don't overheat.

Another highly regulated system is blood pressure with the body making rapid adjustments to try to maintain blood pressure within fairly narrow limits. The body's blood glucose levels are similar. So is water balance, if you get a little bit dehydrated, your body will change a bunch of processes so that you retain water; if you drink a lot of water, you'll pee more to get rid of the excess. On and on it goes and if I sat down and thought about it, probably every other system in your body is equally regulated. So what about body weight?

After three decades of research and endless argument in the journals, it's now well established that human body weight is regulated (it might be more accurate to say that body fat percentage is regulated). Animal studies decades ago demonstrated that the animals would strive to maintain a relatively stable body weight. If you diet them down, they will become less active and slow metabolic rate, rapidly returning to their previous weight when you give them access to food. The same worked in reverse, overfeed them and they will turn off hunger and increase activity rapidly returning to their previous weight.

In humans, studies had demonstrated that metabolism would slow more than you'd predict (for the weight loss) when you dieted people. To a smaller degree, metabolism would also go up when you overfed them. As well, appetite and activity would change accordingly: activity would go down and appetite would go up when people were dieted and activity would tend to increase and appetite would go down when you overfed them. All of which tended to affect body weight/body fat.

In essence, the body is more or less trying to maintain a given level of body fat, that level being called the 'setpoint'. I should mention here that not all scientists agree with the idea of a rigid setpoint, they prefer to think in terms of a settling point, that is a body weight/body fat level that you will settle at depending on circumstances of diet and exercise. This would be roughly equivalent to setting your thermostat higher in the winter and lower in the summer or the cruise control faster on the freeway and slower in town (where the speed limit is lower). You pick a different set(tling) point depending on the circumstances.

So a given individual might settle at one body fat level (and maintain around that level fairly closely) if they were inactive and eating the modern American diet and settle at a different (and generally lower) body fat level if they start exercising and eating better. They would regulate just fine around those settling points (i.e. their body weight would fluctuate a little bit) but they'd have to change habits to alter the settling point very much.

If you think about this within the context of human weight gain, the idea of a settling point is probably a little closer to the truth: people don't continue gaining weight indefinitely. Rather, based on their environment (and, of course genetics), they gain some amount of weight and then stay pretty stable around that new weight. So while you may have weighed a fairly lean 150 in college, when you were active and too poor to afford a lot of food, you stayed around that level of weight. Now that you're older and less active (and can afford more food), you're maintaining at 180 or 200, but you're not continually gaining weight.

Anyhow, the issue of set vs. settling points is sort of tangential to the topic of this chapter. The main idea I want you to take away from this is that within some range, the body appears to 'defend' (another way of saying 'regulate') body weight against change to some degree or another. By 'defend', I mean that it adjusts its physiology to try and maintain that set/settling point within a certain range. Towards this goal, the body can, in premise anyhow, adjust metabolic rate, appetite and a whole host of other systems up or down to try and defend against changes in body fat or body weight.

The physiology of body weight regulation: a (very) brief primer

So let's say you go on a diet, increasing activity or decreasing food intake. Your body senses this and should decrease metabolic rate, increase appetite, decrease activity levels and make fat mobilization and loss more difficult in response. This would make it progressively more difficult to lose weight and easier to regain the lost weight once it was lost. Depending on a host of circumstances, including gender, genetics, and starting body fat percentage (with some others), the body does this pretty well.

Both during a diet as well as afterwards (in what are called the 'post-obese'), metabolic rate tends to be depressed, fat mobilization and burning is decreased, appetite and hunger are increased, and there is a host of other stuff going on. This all serves to make regaining fat after the diet that much easier, something anyone who has fallen off their diet knows all too well: the fat comes on much more rapidly then it came off. I should mention there that this is part of the reason that exercise has been shown to have a greater effect at helping to maintain weight loss than to increase weight (or fat) loss on a diet: exercise helps to offset some of the negative adaptations that occur after weight loss.

In the reverse direction, the body should increase metabolic rate, decrease appetite, increase activity and make fat mobilization easier when you gain weight. However, for reasons discussed in detail in my Bromocriptine book, the system is asymmetrical and most people find it far far easier to gain weight than to lose it. The basic reason, for folks who didn't read that book, being that getting fat was never a problem during our evolutionary past, while starving to death was a very real possibility. So, unlike animals (for whom getting fat means becoming something else's lunch), humans never evolved a good defense against gaining weight. In general, we gain weight pretty easily (as the rapid increase in obesity in the modern world demonstrates) and lose it with more difficulty.

I should mention that a lucky few appear to resist weight gain, their bodies tend to radically increase caloric expenditure and decrease appetite when they start to overeat or gain weight. However, they are in the minority. There is also a group of people who seem to lose weight and fat fairly easily, they too are in the minority.

Depressingly enough, the same people whose bodies resist weight gain the most tend to lose weight the most easily and vice versa: people who find weight loss the most difficult find weight gain relatively easier.

Researchers refer to these as spendthrift (lose weight easily, gain weight with difficulty) and thrifty (lose weight with difficulty, gain weight easily) metabolisms and are busily trying to determine the mechanisms behind the spendthrift metabolism so they can figure out ways to help the thrifty metabolism people. Until the mechanisms behind the different types of metabolism are determined and solutions (which will either require long-term drug intervention or gene therapy) are developed, dieters simply have to accept that some people will have a harder time than others.

How does this work?

Ok, now I don't want to get too deeply into the details of this system, to say it's complicated is an understatement of epic proportion. Rather, I want to sketch the basics since it will be important later in the booklet. The key factors to remember from the thermostat example is that there is a source of input (the temperature), a measurement device (the thermostat/thermometer), and a source of output (in this case, signals to the heater or air conditioner). And, of course, the output then affects the input, forming a loop.

The equivalent of the thermostat in the temperature example above is a part of the brain called the hypothalamus. This is where the body's setpoint is both set and monitored. Sort of tangentially, how the setpoint is set is still being researched. Some of it is assuredly genetic, some people are simply born with a higher setpoint than others. Their bodies regulate body weight normally, they simply do it at a higher level of weight/fat.

There also appear to be critical periods in development, while you were a fetus, immediately after birth, puberty and pregnancy are a few places where the setpoint can change (almost always going up) based on the environment (mainly nutrition and food intake). There is also some evidence that becoming and staying fat can almost permanently raise the setpoint. There is almost no data indicating that the setpoint can ever be brought back down, at least not within any reasonable time span.

Studies of both animals and humans who have maintained weight loss for several years shows no spontaneous recovery of metabolism, it remains slightly depressed. My best guess: if the setpoint ever comes back down, it does so after years and years and years of maintaining a lower weight. In that most people will regain the weight within a few years, this is the same as saying that it never happens.

Anyway, what is the hypothalamus monitoring, what's the source of input? For years, this was the primary question, what was the signal that told the brain what was going on. In 1994, a hormone called leptin was discovered and since then, research has identified a number of hormones within the body that essentially 'tell' the hypothalamus about the current state of your body weight/body fat level. They also inform the hypothalamus about how much you're eating.

These hormones include leptin, insulin, ghrelin, peptide YY, glucose and probably several others (don't worry too much about the names here). The levels of these hormones change when you undereat/lose fat or overeat/gain fat, causing further changes in the levels of various neurochemicals in your brain (the names of which are not important here). Those changes essentially 'tell' your hypothalamus when it's moving away from the setpoint and it takes action.

And what are those actions, that is what's the output? Well, metabolic rate can be adjusted upwards or downwards due to changes in nervous system output and levels of thyroid hormone. Appetite and hunger can change, sometimes drastically. Spontaneous activity can go up or down which is part of why people tend to get lethargic when they diet. Levels of other hormones such as testosterone, estrogen and progesterone can be affected. This is part of why dieting tends to affect women's menstrual cycle and why men who get extremely lean can have problems with libido or sexual function. That's only a partial catalog of the changes that occur.

Those changes further affect body weight and food intake which changes the input and that's how the regulatory loop is formed. This is shown schematically (vastly simplified below.

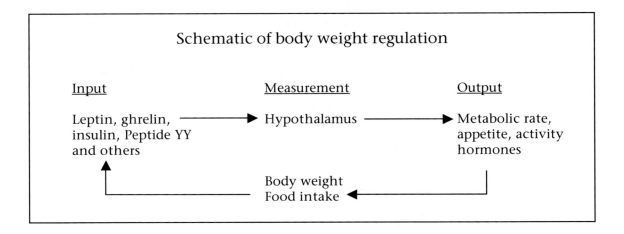

Basically, the brain more or less adjusts the function of the entire body in terms of metabolism, appetite, activity, and hormones when you either under eat or overeat. In general, the response to overeating is the opposite of what happens with under eating: metabolism increases, appetite goes down, spontaneous activity increases, and hormonal status improves.

But, as I mentioned above, the system is not symmetrical and the body is far better at defending against weight loss than weight gain for most people. As well, women tend to better defend against weight loss than men for some rather clear evolutionary reasons (discussed, again, in the Bromocriptine booklet); their bodies fight back harder against diet and exercise programs.

I'm not going to go into much more detail about the system than that, I just wanted readers to have an overview since later chapters dealing with structured refeeds and full diet breaks will make mention of such in terms of how increasing caloric intake can help to fix some of the hormonal problems. In the next chapter, I want to discuss some of the psychological/behavioral reasons why diets fail.

Why Diets Fail Part 2
Introduction

With all of the current research into the biology of body weight regulation (and many other topics related to human genetics), a great many people have started to reach conclusions about body weight being completely biologically determined, how there's nothing we can do about it, hence there's no point in trying in the first place, etc. But, this is an incorrect interpretation of the data.

Now, I could go off on a multipage rant about this topic (genetics versus environment) here but I'll spare you: the key fact to keep in mind is that our biology is never the only determinant of any factor of our biology or behavior. Ok, I take that back, our biology dictates that we will die, it's about the only genetic certainty out there although some researchers think we can even fix that. At most, genetics contribute perhaps 50% (in that range) to any behavior or aspect of our biology. The other 50% (in that range) is environment. As any coach would tell you, the other 90% is mental (little joke there, folks).

Put differently, if you put someone with a high weight/fat 'setpoint' in a third world country where they have to perform daily hard labor and there is little food available, they would not get fat; the environment wouldn't allow it because the food simply isn't available. However, put them in the modern Western environment, with easy access to inexpensive, tasty, high calorie food and low daily activity requirements and they will get fat.

A good (and heavily researched) example of this are the Pima Indians, a group that is divided into roughly two different environments but which share identical genetics. One group of Pima is living the standard Western lifestyle with rather minimal daily activity and easy access to tasty, high-calorie foods; the other is living a much more traditional lifestyle with high levels of daily activity and a more traditional diet. The first group shows a much more extreme prevalence of obesity and Type II diabetes than the second. Once again, it's always genetics plus environment than determine the end result.

That is to say that the biological systems that are trying to pull body weight back to where it was (the 'setpoint') are not deterministic. Human biology works through tendencies and people seem to show varying abilities to resist or act against those tendencies. That is, people clearly do lose weight and successfully keep it off. Are they hungry? Probably. Are their bodies slowing metabolism? Sure. But they simply ignore those signals and control their food intake and increase activity to compensate. Basically, they lose weight and keep it off regardless of the biology that is trying to pull them back to their previous weight. How do they do it? They do it by changing their behavior fairly permanently. Which is basically just a rather long-winded way for me to introduce the next few chapters.

Do diets fail dieters or do dieters fail diets?

As I mentioned before, because of the generally dismal success rates when it comes to dieting, some have even concluded across the board that "Diets don't work". This is only true inasmuch as it ties into the other issues I want to discuss in the following chapters (as well as what I discussed last chapter). That is, realizing that diets fail quite often, we might ask what's failing: the diet or the dieter. Who you ask determines the answer you get.

Generally speaking, the people who are designing and advocating certain diets tend to blame the failure on the dieter. They turn it into a discipline or a laziness issue. Registered dietitians are notorious for this: if their RDA approved diet fails, it's obviously because you cheated. The idea that maybe the diet (or their overall dieting paradigm) is inherently flawed is not even considered.

On the other side, dieters tend to blame the failure on the diet, for a variety of different reasons. Of course, there is some truth to both of the positions and I want to look at both sides of the issue in the next two chapters. As I've mentioned, a diet will continue to work as long as the dieter sticks with it. The question then is why dieters have so much time sticking with diets in the long term, which is what I'm going to address next.

How dieters fail diets

In this chapter, I want to discuss two of the primary ways that dieters tend to sabotage their own efforts on a diet, that is the way that dieters fail diets. These two ways are being too absolute and expecting perfection and by thinking only in the short-term.

And before you complain about how bad it is form wise to write a short introductory paragraph instead of just going straight into the text, I'll defend my style choice by explaining that I don't like starting a chapter with a bold-faced subcategory. So there.

Too absolute/expecting perfection

Perhaps the single biggest reason I have found for dieters failing in their diet effects is that many dieters try to be far too absolute in their approach to the diet something I alluded to in the foreword. When these people are on their diet they are ON THEIR DIET(!!!). Which is altogether fine as long as they stay on the diet. The problem is that any slip, no matter how small, is taken as complete and utter failure. The diet is abandoned and the post-diet food binge begins. As I've mentioned, this tends to put the fat (and frequently a little extra) back on faster than before.

We have all either known (or been) the following person: one cookie eaten in a moment of weakness or distraction, the guilt sets in, and the rest of the bag is GONE (perhaps inhaled is the proper word). Anything worth doing is worth overdoing, right? Psychologists refer to such individuals as rigid dieters, they see the world in a rather extreme right or wrong approach, either they are on their diet, and 100% perfection is expected, or they are off their diet, shoveling crap in as fast as it will go. I'm quite sure this type of attitude is not limited to dieting, probably any behavior you care to name finds people at one extreme or the other.

As a side note, you can oftentimes see the same attitude with people starting an exercise program. The first few weeks go great, workouts are going well, then a single workout is missed. The person figures that any benefits are lost because of missing that one workout and they never go back to the gym.

Now, I could probably go on for pages about this one topic but I'll spare you the verbiage. My main point out that there are times (most of them) when obsessive dedication or the expectation of perfection becomes a very real source of failure. Sure, if it drives you towards better and better results, such an attitude will work. But only until you finally slip. Note that I said 'until you slip' not 'if you slip'. In most cases, it's a matter of when, not if you're going to break your diet.

If you take the attitude that anything less than absolute perfection is a failure, you're pretty much doomed from the start. Now, there are some exceptions, places where results have to obtained in a very short time frame and you can't really accept mistakes. Athletes who have a short time to get to a certain level of body fat or muscle mass, for whom victory or defeat may hinge on their ability to suffer for long enough are one. I mentioned some others in The Rapid Fat Loss Handbook, situations where individuals need or want to reach some drastic goal in a very short period of time; even there I included some deliberate breaks for both psychological and physiological reasons. But in the grand majority of cases, this type of obsessive, no-exceptions attitude tends to cause more problems that it solves.

Keeping with this idea, psychologists frequently talk about something called the 80/20 principle which says that 'If you're doing what you're supposed to do 80% of the time, the other 20% doesn't matter'. While there are certainly exceptions (try avoiding crack or heroin for 80% of the time), it certainly applies to dieting and exercise under the grand majority of conditions.

If the changes you've made to your diet and exercise program stay solid for 80% of the time, the other 20% is no big deal. Not unless you make it one. And that's really the issue, that 20% problem only becomes one if the dieter decides (either consciously or unconsciously) to make it a problem. Once again, the exception is for those folks under strict time frames, who don't have the option to screw up. For everyone else, seeking perfection means seeking failure.

Focusing only on the short-term

The second primary way that dieters fail diets is focusing only on the short-term and this applies in a couple of different ways. The first is a reality issue. Ignoring diets promising quick, easy weight loss (my Rapid Fat Loss Handbook caused rapid weight loss, a great deal of which was water, but it sure isn't easy), about the best you can usually do with true fat loss is somewhere between 1.5-3 lbs./week (fatter individuals can sometimes lose more).

Sure you can drop a lot more total weight if you factor in water weight and other contributors but true fat loss typically peaks at about that rate (some lighter women may have trouble even losing one pound of fat per week).

For the sake of example, let's say 2 lbs./week can be reasonably expected for a fatter individual. For someone with a large amount of fat to lose, 50 or 100 pounds, this may mean one-half to a full year of dieting. Possibly more since it's rare to see perfectly linear fat loss without stalls or plateaus.

Consider the reality of that, you may have to alter eating and exercise habits for nearly a year just to reach your goal. Do you really expect to be hungry and deprived for that entire period? I thought not. If you have a lot of weight/fat to lose, you need to start thinking in the long-term, you will need to make changes to diet or activity (or both) and maintain them in the long-term.

As a second issue: a lot of dieters seem to think that once they have lost the weight with one diet or another, they can revert to their old habits and keep the weight off. So they change their eating habits drastically, drop the weight and then go right back to the way of eating that made them fat. And, to their apparent surprise, they get fat again. "You can never go back again." as the old saying goes. If you go back to the diet and exercise habits that made you fat in the first place, you'll just get fat again.

This actually makes a profound argument for making small, livable changes to your eating and activity habits and avoiding the type of extreme approach that I described in my last booklet. The simple reason being that small changes seem to be easier to maintain in the long-term, even if they don't generate results as rapidly. And that's actually sort of the tradeoff, the types of small changes that tends to be sustainable in the long-term tend to cause weight/fat loss that is so painfully slow (or minimal) as to be almost irrelevant; and the types of extreme approaches that generate rapid results tend to be nearly impossible to stick to in the long-term. A potential compromise, and one I addressed somewhat in The Rapid Fat Loss Handbook is using an extreme diet (such as the one described in that booklet) to generate initial rapid weight/fat losses and then move into a more traditional or moderate diet for the longer term.

At the end of the day, here's the painful reality that all dieters must come to terms with: the only way to both lose fat AND maintain that loss in the long-term is to maintain at least some of the diet and exercise habits you changed in the long-term. Forever, basically even though that's a little too depressing to consider. Maybe we should just think long-term instead. Hopefully we'll get genetic engineering soon enough to make it a not-forever kind of deal.

Dieters (or anyone seeking to change a long-standing behavior) must stop thinking of diets as a short-term behavior change, you'll have to maintain at least some of those changes in the long-term. Now, I'll point out here that the strategies used for weight/fat loss and maintenance aren't necessarily going to be the same (nor should they be). As I talked about in the Rapid Fat Loss Handbook, there are situations where an extreme diet can be used initially and used to move into a proper maintenance phase. A lot of diet researchers and diet book authors miss this point, thinking that the diet that you followed to lose the weight/fat must or should be the same as the one you use to maintain that loss.

I do think it's helpful is the diet that caused the fat loss can be used to move into a maintenance approach (again, something I discussed in some detail in the last booklet and will make mention of in this one) but they needn't be the same. If eliminating all of the carbohydrates from your diet makes it easier to lose fat in the long run, and you are able to move back to a maintenance diet that contains some carbohydrates, I don't see what the problem is. Once again, the diet you use to lose the fat doesn't necessarily have to be the same diet as you use to maintain that fat loss. If nothing else, you get to eat more when you move back to maintenance, the types of foods you allow yourself may change as well.

Summing up this section, it's not that diets per se fail, it's that diets that are only followed short-term fail. The body is really good at storing incoming calories as fat after a diet and if you return to old eating habits, you can just watch the pounds come flying back on.

To hopefully cement this point in your mind, studies of successful dieters (those who have lost weight and kept it off for some period of time, usually 2-5 years) have shown several very consistent behavior patterns of which this is one: they maintain the dietary and exercise changes they have made in the long-term. If you're not going to maintain at least some of your changed dietary and exercise habits in the long-term, you might as well not bother (with one major exception discussed below).

One exception to what I wrote above

There is, however, one major exception to the above that I should probably mention (and that I discuss in greater detail in my Rapid Fat Loss Handbook). There are individuals who, for whatever reason, only have to be in shape for a very short period of time, a day or three at the most, who don't necessarily care if the results are maintained long-term or not.

Usually it's a bodybuilder preparing for a contest, or even a model who has a particularly important photo shoot. Or a woman who needs to drop 20 lbs. for her wedding or a male who wants to impress people at his high school reunion. Even athletes who have to make a weight class sometimes have to do scary stuff to get where they need to be, usually involving fluid restriction and frequently severe dehydration. But the consequences of not making weight (whatever they may be) are greater than the extreme approaches that tend to be used.

In situations like that, whether it's healthy or not, extremely restrictive and/or even slightly dangerous approaches are frequently used. We may not like them, we may not condone them but sometimes the ends justifies the means because a few pounds may mean the difference in getting a big paycheck/winning the contest/looking good in your wedding gown or not.

In these situations, long-term maintenance isn't necessarily the goal. No sane bodybuilder expects to maintain contest shape year-round, and no weight class athlete expects to maintain a severe state of dehydration year round. They get in shape for their event, and relax to some degree for the rest of the time. So the above sections really are aimed at the person looking to lose fat and keep it off long-term.

In that case, where maintenance is just as important as the loss itself, absolute attitudes and focusing only on the short-term hurt far more than they help, and should be avoided as much as possible. In addition to the strategies I'm going to discuss in this booklet, this means taking a very different attitude towards dieting. First you have to let go of your absolutist attitudes, which can be hard. Second, you need to start taking the long view to both your weight loss and dietary and exercise habits. I'll come back to this in later chapters.

How diets fail dieters

Yes, another short waste of space paragraph to introduce this chapter. If you don't like my writing style, feel free to write your own book. In the last chapter, I discussed the two major ways that dieters tend to fail diets, by being too absolute and expecting perfection and by focusing only on the short-term. In this chapter, I want to discuss the ways that diets themselves can be the problem: by causing too much hunger, and by not being matched to the dieter.

Too much hunger

One of the biggest causes of diet failure is plain old hunger. It's no coincidence that the majority of diet pills are appetite suppressants (others increase metabolic rate or decrease the number of calories absorbed from the stomach). It started with amphetamines in the 50's and went from there. Phen/Fen was one of the most recent diet drugs with newer compounds like Meridia and others being used more currently. The much maligned ephedrine/caffeine stack partly works by suppressing hunger (it also increases metabolic rate and fat burning).

By decreasing or reducing appetite through chemical means, these types of drugs cause weight loss. Since nearly all of them are stimulants of some sort, most of them have side effects and/or can't be used in the long-term. And most will eventually quit working as the body adapts, unless you keep increasing the dosages. Unless they are used along with changes to diet and exercise habits, any weight loss effects are purely short-term anyhow.

By extension, a good long-term diet should do at least some job of controlling appetite. Many diets fail in this regards. Part of the problem is that human appetite is brutally complex and every new piece of research only adds to the complexity of the system (the chapter on body weight regulation addressed this very briefly). This is a topic where a book should and could be written. Yeah I know, get on it Lyle. One of these days. For now just accept that it's really complicated.

Human appetite is regulated by an incredibly complex number of biological systems including but not limited to: the physical stretching of the stomach, the levels of different nutrients in the blood, brain chemistry, and even changes in fat cell size. Humans are also one of the few animals who eat for purely non-hunger related reasons. These include boredom, depression, because it's meal time, because we saw a tv commercial for something tasty on, because we are out with friends, etc.

Anorexics may continue to starve themselves in the face of massive hunger while people who are full to the point of being sick may continue eating at Thanksgiving or an all you can eat buffet simply because the food is there and they don't want to let it 'go to waste'. Basically, there is a complex interaction of both physiological and psychological components to human eating behavior and it's the interaction that determines the end results.

As if it weren't complicated enough, people seem to vary in what types of foods and diet setups will control their appetite. Individuals with severe insulin resistance, hyperinsulinemia and rebound hypoglycemia (low blood sugar) may get rebound hunger from even small amounts of carbohydrates in their diet, others may fill up on a slice of bread or two. Some people have their appetite almost blocked completely by low-carbohydrate/ketogenic diets. Others have no such luck, and overeat because of the high dietary fat content that can occur with such diets.

Without going off on one of my typical rants, this is one of the huge problems I have with any diet book claiming to have THE ANSWER (TM), that any single diet can possibly be appropriate for all individuals under all circumstances. Outside of every other important issue, human appetite and hunger is simply too complex for a single diet to control them in every situation. This gets into the topic of the next section, that the diet must be matched to the dieter.

Even with that said, it would be a rare diet indeed that completely blocked appetite forever. A lot of people bitch (a lot) about having to restrict their food intake. It's no fun but that's the price you pay: you can either suck it up or stay fat. Those are your choices. Even athletes and bodybuilders, who should be prepared to suffer for their sport, will complain in this respect. And it's not just psychological weakness. Changes in brain chemistry, under the influence of signals from other parts of your body, are sending powerful 'eat now!' signals to you as you starve your body into submission.

And again, that's just physiology. As I mentioned above, there's another important aspect to human eating behavior: the psychological aspect. Think about what would happen if someone told you you could NEVER eat a certain food again. Not just a little while, not a month or three, but NEVER. Assuming it wasn't a food you hated to begin with (brussel sprouts anyone?), you'd start to crave that food. Eventually, you would probably binge on it. For no other reason than knowing you couldn't have it. It's simple human nature: we want what we can't have. At a lesser extreme, simply knowing that you can't eat when and what you want tends to make people anxious and hungry.

The idea that a diet can be too restrictive or too absolute goes hand in hand with what was discussed in the previous chapter. On top of dieters enforcing ridiculous amounts of food restriction themselves and expecting absolute perfection, many diets go even further in restricting food options.

Now sometimes this is a necessity that really can't be worked around. High sugar carbohydrates have to be pretty much restricted on diabetic or ketogenic diets, the PSMF described in The Rapid Fat Loss Handbook mandated specific foods as it was trying to minimize caloric intake while ensuring essential nutrient intake. Point being that it's hard to design a diet that lets people eat everything they want whenever they want; that's what folks are doing now and all it's doing is making them fat.

Additionally, some people seem to have what approaches food addictions regarding certain foods (or categories of food), these are sometimes called trigger foods. If those folks eat even a little of their trigger food, they will eat a ton of it. Clearly, in that situation, complete avoidance (or very controlled intake) is the only solution. But in most cases, you can generally find happy compromises. To one degree, the flexible dieting concepts I'm going to talk about very shortly solve this problem entirely anyhow.

Not matched to the dieter

Although there are exceptions, the grand majority of diets out there are fairly simple one-size-fits-all approaches, something I mentioned briefly above. Yes, there may be some slight individualization (usually in terms of protein intake or calories but sometimes not even that) but for the most part, diet book authors tend to take a one diet for all people approach. The majority of mainstream nutritionists and RDs take the same attitude. To say that I find this approach absurd is an understatement.

Although humans share the same general physiology, there are always subtle differences. Any physician knows that the drug that will work optimally for one person may not work as well for another, even if they suffer from the same disease. This is why there are different drug options for different diseases.

You find the same thing in exercise programs. While there are certainly general principles that apply to just about everyone, there is most also certainly variance in what people respond to. It's not as simple as saying 'Do this and ye shall succeed' or a lot more people would be succeeding. Some individualization is always needed.

Of course, this makes it very difficult to write a diet book since people tend to like having simple answers handed to them on a platter. It's a big part of why I haven't written the diet book I want to write yet, trying to factor in all the considerations I make in setting up a diet for someone and putting it into a coherent book form has been too much of a hassle to this point. The next to last chapter of both The Rapid Fat Loss Handbook and this book is my rough attempt to put some of my thoughts on the topic down, one of these days I'll get off my lazy butt and put them all down in one monster diet book.

Anyhow, for some reason, both diet book authors and RD's are too arrogant (or too stupid) to realize that the same principle applies to diets: there can't be any single approach that works for all people or all situations equally well. Of course, it takes less thought on the part of the person giving the diet advice (and makes writing diet books much easier). This type of approach also appeals more to the American public. They want to be given THE ANSWER (TM) and not have to think too much about it beyond that.

Of course, when you consider the miserable results statistics of those same groups (slim and none with obesity getting worse not better), you start to realize that it's not working. And I have a rather simple rule: if something isn't working, you change it.

A brief tangent: A few words about diet

Now, I don't intend to talk in that much detail about the different diets that are out there in this booklet; the principles of flexible dieting I'm going to discuss can be applied to any diet out there as far as I'm concerned. As necessary, I will make specific comments in the individual chapters on the flexible dieting strategies and how different diets might apply them. For now, I'll only say that a fat loss diet needs to meet a few basic requirements.

The first is that it has to cause an imbalance between your energy expenditure (via daily activity and exercise) and your energy intake (from food). As I mentioned previously, even diets that tell you you don't have to count or restrict calories will trick you into doing it anyhow. They'll simply give you a set of rules on what and when you can eat that will tend to make overeating more difficult. I do the same, and discussed this topic in more detail in the (now, altogether too often mentioned) Rapid Fat Loss Handbook as well as in this book.

For example, since fat is calorie dense (contains a lot of calories in a little bit of space), low-fat diets tend to cause people to eat less, at least initially. Then they invariably start eating more of the foods that they are allowed and weight loss stops or reverses.

Low-carbohydrate diets work, to a great degree, the same way. When you make people remove a category of foods that probably makes up a majority of their daily calories, they can't help but eat less. Of course, they too usually end up eating too much over time, increasing their intake of allowed foods such that weight loss stalls or reverses.

The same goes for any other diet you care to name: they may use different methods of doing it but one way or another, they cause a skew in how many calories you're taking in relative to what you're burning. And they all more or less work, at least in the short-term.

A second requirement as far as I'm concerned is adequate protein and recent research is finally catching up to what smart athletes and bodybuilders have known for decades: diets that are higher in protein (at least 25% of total calories) work better then diets lower in protein. There are a number of reasons for this, one of them being that protein is the most appetite blunting nutrient; people who eat more protein tend to eat less calories and stay full longer. As well, diets higher in protein tend to cause slightly more fat loss and slightly less LBM loss. Additionally, higher protein intakes stabilize blood glucose compared to higher carbohydrate intakes which helps to stabilize energy levels as well as hunger. Bottom line, get plenty of protein, preferably from leaner sources like chicken, fish, low-fat meats. Dairy calcium is turning out to have some nice benefits in terms of health and fat loss so a source of dairy protein (milk or yogurt for carb based diets, cheeses of varying sorts for low-carb diets) is also a good idea.

A good diet should also contain plenty of roughage, vegetables (and some fruits, noting that fruits can be surprisingly high in calories sometimes) which goes a long way in keeping you full. Additionally, some provision for essential fatty acids (the fish oils that the media keeps talking about) should be made. Some studies have found that moderate fat intakes show better adherence, especially compared to very low-fat diets (which tend to taste like cardboard).

Frankly, beyond those few requirements, I feel that the rest of the diet has more to do with what's appropriate for the individual than anything else. Folks doing more high intensity exercise tend to need more carbohydrates than those who are not. Folks who are insulin resistant seem to do better (both from a diet and health perspective) when they reduce carbohydrates. A recent paper reached the 'brilliant' conclusion that the best diet for weight loss is the one that people will stick to (this is something I've been saying for years). Within some range, it's as much about finding a diet that you can live with in the long-term as anything else.

I will say that in general, people who feel great on carb based diets tend to do poorly and and feel horrible on low-carbohydrate diets, they feel lethargic and listless. By the same token, individuals who find that their energy levels crash badly on carbohydrate based diets tend to do well and feel great when they reduce carbohydrates and increase protein, fat and fiber.

Again, this booklet isn't my fat loss/diet book so I'm not going to get into much more detail than this (I have an article or two on my website if you want to delve into it a bit more). I'll only say that if you're on a particular popular diet and you feel terrible, with low energy and such, you should try something else. Regardless of whatever convincing bit of science (or, as is so often the case, pseudoscience) the author fed you, if you feel terribly or aren't losing weight it clearly isn't working for you and you have nothing to lose by trying something else.

Summary

So there's a basic overview of some of the reasons I think diets tend to fail dieters, although I'm sure I've left one or two contributors out. I'll merely say that those are the ones that I think are most relevant to this booklet. And, ignoring the issue of the diet simply not fitting the dieter's needs, all of the other issues basically come down to the problem with either the diet requiring an insane amount of restriction and deprivation, or the dieter enforcing it upon themselves. In both cases, the cause is essentially the same. In both cases, the solution happens to be the same: flexible dieting.

Introduction to Flexible Dieting

Now that you have a better idea why, in my opinion anyhow, most diets tend to fail, I'd like to finally introduce you to the flexible dieting concepts of this booklet. You may already have a reasonable idea from reading the previous chapters but just in case (and to pad out the length of this booklet), I want to go into a few more details in this chapter. Then, after another tangent chapter where I have you get a rough estimate of your current body fat percentage, I'll introduce you to the three different types of flexible dieting concepts and explain how to integrate them.

What is flexible dieting?

As the name suggests, and the last chapters sort of implied, the basic idea of flexible dieting is that you aren't expecting absolute perfection and strictness in your dieting behavior. Rather, small (or even larger) lapses from your diet simply aren't any big deal in the big scheme of things.

Once again, let's put dieting into perspective here. Let's say that you have enough fat to lose that you may be dieting for one half to one year straight. Let's say that you've been absolutely great on your diet for the last 4-5 days or even the last few weeks. Now you come up against one of those situations that I mentioned in the foreword.

Say you eat that single cookie. In the big scheme of things, what's the big deal, really? So you had 100 calories extra from that cookie. Within the context of the period of proper eating (proper means following whatever diet you're on), that 100 calories is simply no big deal. Now, if you take that 100 calorie lapse as an excuse to eat the entire bag, to the tune of 1000 calories, you've just taken what is no big deal and made it into one.

Or let's look at a slightly different perspective. Say you've been on your diet just perfectly for the last 4-5 days (or longer). Now you get a craving for something sweet. Those cookies are calling but you're afraid that the one cookie is going to blow your entire diet. You resist and resist and resist until finally you give in and, because of the huge cravings you've now generated, you end up eating the whole bag. Which generates the same, if not more, guilt to boot and you throw your diet out the window. That's an example of the types of rigid dieting that tends to derail dieting efforts. Contrast that to changing your mental attitude: you want a cookie, you have one cookie, you realize that it's no big deal in the big scheme of things, you deal with the craving before it gets out of hand and then get on with your life. The latter attitude would be consistent with flexible dieting.

Or say you've been dieting and you've got a special even coming up. A birthday, a dinner party, whatever. Now, if you're still in the rigid mindset, you'll either go to the party and be miserable because you don't get to eat any of the good stuff or you'll decide that your diet is clearly blown and go off of it completely and shovel as much crap down your throat as you possibly can.

Again, let's look at the long-term perspective: can a single meal really be that relevant to your overall diet (again, remember that you may have one half to a full year of dieting to reach your goal)? Of course not. If you've been following your diet properly for the past 4-5 days (or weeks or whatever), that single meal is simply no big deal. Unless you make it into one.

A flexible dieter would realize that that single meal is no big deal, go enjoy themselves at the party and get on with their life. They might try to limit their intake (don't go have 4 pieces of cake or anything like that) at the party or even earlier in the day but they would still enjoy themselves at the party.

Consider the final example from the foreword, a situation where you have an extended period where following your diet will be more difficult. Perhaps it's a family vacation, a cruise, something along those lines. Holidays always tend to be miserable times for dieters, with regular parties and an extended period where it's nearly impossible to keep on your diet.

There actually a couple of workable approaches to this type of situation. One is to simply do the best you can, damage control if it were. Even if you maintain your current diet for most of the time (even if it's only 2 meals out of 3), that's still better than blowing your diet and shoveling down as much crap as you can at every meal, right? But that's not the only option here; there's a second option I'm going to describe next.

The diet didn't fail but science did: The importance of control

Before I continue, I want to tell you about one of the coolest studies I've seen in a while. I say cool mainly because of the fact that the scientists failed so miserably in their goal, while making an absolutely wonderful discovery. For anybody who wants to look it up, the full reference is "Wing RR and RW Jeffrey. Prescribed 'Breaks' as a means to disrupt weight control efforts. Obes Res (2003) 11: 287-291."

The study was set up to find out why people go off the dieting bandwagon. That is, the researchers wanted to determine what behavioral things happen when people go off of their diet for some period, and why they have trouble going back on.

So the subjects were first put on a typical diet meant to cause weight loss. Then the subjects were told to go off the diet for either 2 weeks or 6 weeks so that the researchers could see what happened when people fell off their diet but hard and started regaining weight. Here's what happened: not only did the subjects not regain very much weight, but they had almost no trouble going right back onto their diet when the 2 (or 6) weeks was over. So the scientists completely and utterly failed to reach their goal of studying what they wanted to study.

Basically, they made an almost accidental discovery which raised another set of questions: why didn't the subjects regain a ton of weight and why did they have little problem returning to their diet? That is, knowing that most people who go off of a diet for even a short period will balloon up, regaining weight rapidly, and fall off their diet, what made this study (or these subjects) different?

The basic issue seemed to come down to that of control. To understand this, let's consider two different situations. First let's say that you're the typical rigid dieter hammering away on your perfect diet, no lapses, no mistakes. Suddenly something comes up that is out of your control. A stressful period of life, the aforementioned vacation, whatever. Feeling out of control, you figure your diet is blown and the binge begins. Does this sound familiar at all?

But consider what happened in this study, the subjects were told by the researchers to go off their diet; in essence, the break was part of the diet. And they didn't blow up, didn't gain a ton of weight, and had no problem going right back onto the diet.

I suspect that that was the key difference and why the study failed so miserably: control. Psychologically, feeling like the break is now under your control, or that it's part of your overall plan, makes it far easier to not feel like the diet is completely blown and get back on the diet when things settle down. Which brings me to one more word of introduction.

Flexible dieting: Planned or unplanned

I think some people are able to be flexible dieters without hugely specific plans but I'm not sure this is the case universally. This is especially true for rigid dieters who are trying to adopt flexible dieting attitudes. My concern is that people will use the flexible dieting concepts I've presented so far in this booklet as an excuse to break their diet a little too frequently and I don't think that will work either. Losing weight still requires that you diet, I'm simply trying to make you understand that expecting yourself to adhere to your diet 100% without exception is generally a recipe for disaster.

That is, it's a little too easy to say, on a daily basis "I really need this cookie (or three) and I'm being a flexible" dieter, and Lyle the diet guru said it was ok. But that's not going to cut it either. Instead, in a couple of chapters, I'm going to present a scheme where you plan to break your diet (for varying amounts of time depending on the circumstance) based on your current body fat percentage.

So rather than let your diet breaks fall where they may (although there may be situations where this is unavoidable), I think having a bit of control over them, at least at first, will be the most useful. With time, you may be able to diet successfully and apply the flexible dieting a little more spontaneously. But, if you're the typical rigid dieter trying it a different way, I think it's a better to make things sort of a rigid flexible dieting approach (for what sense that makes) in the initial stages.

A case study on flexible dieting: My mom

Ok, I want to make it clear that I dislike diet books that throw testimonials at readers, for the simple fact that it's far too easy to pick and choose from super successful folks and to ignore failures (who typically quit using the diet anyhow). Basically, I consider the use of those kinds of testimonials to be a little disingenuous in the first place. So in presenting my mom's experience with the concepts I'm talking about in this book, I want to make it clear that they are meant to be as an example only. I offer it not as proof of the concepts I'm describing but a real-world example of how someone applied them.

My mom, as is the case with most dieters, has ridden the standard diet rollercoaster for quite some time. While certainly not fat, she has carried perhaps 30 pounds of extra weight with most of that coming after menopause. Diets, for her, were generally an all or nothing affair moving from one extreme of another. Several years back, and I'm not sure how much my badgering of her had to do with this, her attitude seemed to change. One way or another, she started to adopt what turned out to be flexible dieting concepts.

Last year for example, she got involved with the Weight Watchers programs (one of the few commercial diet programs that I think is worth a crap). At one point in her diet, it turned out that she had a three-day trip to New York, a situation similar to what I described in the foreword and above. Now, you'd be crazy to think that she was going to go to NY and not enjoy herself food wise. The friend she was going with asked "So does that mean that you're off your diet?" Mom told her no, that she was simply going to enjoy herself over the weekend, not worry about it, and get right back on the program when she got back into town. Which is exactly what she did. She went to NY and enjoyed herself. She didn't gain any (significant) amount of weight over the weekend and had no problem returning to her diet that following Monday.

As a longer term example (similar to the study I described above), every summer for the past many years, mom goes to Europe to play piano. Now, food in Europe tends to be notoriously fatty (especially where my mom is) so there's only so much that she can do in terms of sticking to her normal diet. But rather than worry overly about it, she does her best (it also helps that she walks everywhere which ends up burning off a lot of the excess calories) food wise. When she gets back to the states, she has had no trouble taking off any slight weight that she gained.

There are other examples of places my mom has adopted a flexible dieting mentality; for example, if she wants a little something sweet, she'll have it and move on with her life. She's finally realized that a tiny bit now is better than bingeing later because she felt deprived and that that small bit of sweets (or what have you) is no big deal in the big

30

scheme of things. And her success at maintaining her weight loss has been much higher this time around.

Again, this singular example isn't meant to prove anything. I'm presenting it simply as an example of the types of mental shifts I'm trying to describe in this booklet: how relaxing your expectations of both yourself and your diet can be far more productive for your long-term dieting success than the converse. Nothing more and nothing less.

Determining your body fat percentage

I didn't just introduce you to the concept of body fat versus body weight in chapter two to bore you or to lengthen this booklet to justify the cost (ok, that wasn't entirely the reason). So why did I bother to make the distinction?

One reason is that tracking changes in body fat percentage is a relatively more accurate measure of what's going on with your diet than just tracking weight. For example, if you start a diet and exercise program, it's not uncommon to lose body fat while gaining muscle weight; this means that your body weight may not change (making you think that your diet isn't working) but your body fat percentage is going down. However, after writing that whole long paragraph for you to read, I'm not going to give you a method that really allows that here.

For the purposes of this booklet, the main reason to really have any idea of what your body fat percentage is is that it will determine how you utilize the three different types of flexible dieting I'm going to describe in the next chapters. Of course, you can use the method I'm going to describe to track changes to some degree. Just be aware of the qualifications I'm going to make below regarding this method.

Estimating body fat percentage

There are a number of methods of estimating body fat percentage (note my use of the word 'estimating'; that's all it is, an estimate) ranging from lo-tech to high-tech and accurate to horribly inaccurate. Which you use depends on your goals and what you have access to. I won't bore you listing all of them, rather I'll focus on which ones I think are worth pursuing in this specific case.

Relatively lean individuals, athletes or bodybuilders, should either know what their body fat percentage is or have some reasonable method of estimating it. Calipers would be my preferred method. If you know about calipers, I don't need to give you any more information. If you don't, it won't do me any good to explain them here so I'm not going to.

Another possible method, although fraught with potential problems are the bioelectrical impedance body fat scales (Tanita is a common brand). The problem is that these devices are drastically affected by hydration, a large glass of water or a big piss can alter the number. In general, I don't think they are that accurate but assuming you control for hydration, they can at least give you a starting point and some ability to track relative changes.

Now, what about everybody else? Frankly, if you're not that lean and not currently very active, there's a fairly easy way to get a rough estimate of your body fat percentage and that is by using something called the Body Mass Index (BMI). BMI is supposed to be a measure of fatness but it's really not, what it does is relate height and weight with certain BMI ranges (supposedly) being associated with health or not. The problem with BMI is that it doesn't factor body fat percentage into account.

That is, say we have two individuals who are 6 feet tall and weigh 200 lbs.. But say one is an athlete and has 10% body fat and the other is not and has 30% body fat. They will have the same BMI value but it's fairly clear (it should be anyhow) that they are not going to be in the same boat in terms of health risk or anything else. Basically, BMI makes no distinction between fat mass and LBM and since active individuals typically have more LBM (and hence less fat) at any given body weight, BMI is not accurate for them.

However, recent research allows us to use BMI to get a *rough* idea of body fat percentage. Since we're not looking for exacting numbers, it's ok. But I must repeat: active individuals MUST find a different method (i.e. calipers or a Tanita scale or something) to estimate body fat, they can NOT use the BMI method.

Determining BMI

To save everyone a bunch of calculations, I've made determining BMI as easy as looking at the chart in Appendix 1. All you need to know is your height and scale weight. Since I know that many of my readers are probably used to the metric system, I've included both metric (weight in kilograms, height in meters) and American (weight in pounds, height in feet and inches) values. Simply cross-reference your weight and height and find your BMI on the table. If you fall in-between values, just pick the middle value. Once again, we're not concerned with exacting accuracy, just a general idea. Once you've determined your BMI, use table 2 in Appendix 1 to get a rough estimate of your body fat percentage.

Putting the number to use

In my last booklet, I had readers use their estimated body fat percentage to determine their fat mass and lean body mass since I had them using their LBM value to set up the diet in terms of protein intake. In this booklet, I still want you to go ahead and estimate your body fat percentage and estimate LBM as well. First you're going to multiply your current weight (either in pounds or kilograms) by your body fat percentage (divide the percentage by 100 so 30% becomes 0.30) to determine how much of your total weight is fat.

```
_____ * _____ = _____
Weight   BF%      Total fat
```

Now subtract the pounds of fat from your total weight, this is how much LBM you have.

```
_____ - _____ = _____
Total weight   Total fat    LBM
```

Next, I want you to use Table 1 on the next page to determine what dieting category you are in (1, 2 or 3) based on your current body fat percentage.

Please note that, to a degree, the separation between these categories is arbitrary, it would be more accurate to put them on a continuum. However, for ease of use, I have to make the divisions somewhere and this is where they fall. If you're right on the edge of a category, it's probably best to use the lower category. So a male who came in at 26% body fat should consider themselves in Category 2, rather than Category 3.

Every so often, you will probably want to re-determine your estimated body fat percentage, as some of my recommendations regarding refeeds and the full diet break will change. If you're right on the edge of categories, you can probably check again a few weeks into your diet; if it's not totally retarded, you have probably dropped down a category. If not, checking for changes every 4-8 weeks is generally sufficient.

Table 1: Determining diet category based on body fat percentage

Category	Male BF%	Female BF%
1	15% and lower	24% and lower
2	16-25%	25-34%
3	26%+	35%+

In the next several chapters, I'm going to introduce you to the three different components of flexible dieting: free meals, structured refeeds, and full diet breaks. Based on your current body fat percentage, each one will have relatively more or less applicability and I'll discuss each within the context of that category so keep it in mind.

I'm also going to make a few comments about how you might utilize the different flexible dieting approaches based on what type of weight/fat loss diet you're currently on. Since I can't cover every possible diet (there are thousands of them out there), I'm going to assume that my readers are either using some form of high-carbohydrate/low-fat diet, a Zone/Isocaloric type of diet (where the ratios of protein, carbs and fat are fairly close to one another) or some type of low-carbohydrate diet (such as an Atkins, Protein Power or South Beach type of diet). Once again, while this won't cover everybody, it should cover the majority.

Estimating your activity level

Although it's sort of out of place for this chapter, I couldn't think of anywhere else to include this section. Now that you have estimated your body fat percentage and determined your dieting category and LBM level, I want you to make a rough estimate of your current activity (exercise) level. In my last booklet, I separated folks into three categories but in this one I'm only going to use two.

You are in exercise Category 1 if you are performing some type of weight training a minimum of 2-3 times per week for an hour or so. I'm not talking about just waving around little baby pink weights either, I mean real weight training. Category 1 also includes endurance athletes such as runners or cyclists who are either doing fairly long workouts (1-4 hours at a decent intensity) or intensive workouts (near lactate threshold or above). If you don't know what the term lactate threshold means, you're most likely not exercising anywhere close to it, put yourself in Category 2.

If you're only performing low-intensity aerobic exercise, or just moving around baby weights in the weight room or doing no exercise at all, you're in exercise Category 2.

Free meals

The first flexible dieting concept I want to describe is the free meal. Some people call this a cheat meal but others find the word 'cheat' has too many negative connotations and puts them back into a negative mindset. Reward meal is another typical description with a few diet approaches allowing a single 'reward' meal per day or so (for example The Carbohydrate Addicts Diet by the Hellers).

Just as it sounds, this is a single meal that breaks your diet. When I say break I mean that it doesn't conform to the rest of the diet in either the amount or types of foods you get to eat. So someone on a low-carbohydrate diet might eat those high carb, high-starch foods (bread, pasta, and the like) that they've been craving. Someone on a low-fat diet might have those French fries or pizza or something greasy. Someone on a Zone type of diet would simply eat without worrying about achieving some specific ratio of nutrients. The main thing is that the free meal lets you address any cravings you might have by allowing you to have a little of those 'forbidden' foods.

The main benefit of the free meal is simply psychological; a single meal isn't really long enough to affect the various hormones (leptin, ghrelin, etc.) that are involved in the physiological response to dieting. Dieting nonstop for extended periods on end gets to be a real mental grind. Knowing that there is light at the end of the tunnel, that a couple of times per week you can eat more or less 'freely' goes a long way in keeping your sanity.

This tends to help with long-term adherence since you never suffer from the psychologically induced deprivation that you can't EVER have a certain food. You know that you're never more than a few days away from a free meal which makes those days of dieting far more tolerable. Also, if you have any sort of a social life (family or dating), a free meal gives you the ability to eat with everybody else without being a huge pain in the ass.

The first obligatory warning: how NOT to do a free meal

I've learned through experience that people tend to read very selectively, they'll read until they see what they want to see and then stop (a friend calls this a cafeteria approach to reading). Which means that putting warnings at the end of the chapter, after I've told you the good stuff tends to cause problems. Instead, you get the warnings before the information so you can't claim that you just happened to stop reading and didn't see what I'm about to say.

So, before you stop reading and go out and start gorging, let's talk about what a free meal is and is not. A free meal is NOT a deliberate attempt to see how much food you can stuff down your gullet in a single meal although this is how it is all too commonly interpreted. The problem I all too often see is that people fall out of one psychological trap (that breaking the diet at all is a huge failure on their part) and into another (they try to see how much crap they can gorge themselves on during their breaks). Both cause problems. So don't decide that you're going to try and put down the entire pizza (or two), or bankrupt the all you can eat buffet on your free meal; that's a complete and utter abuse of what the free meal is supposed to accomplish.

Rather, go eat a 'normal' meal where you are not supremely obsessed with the content. Don't get me wrong, striving to make healthier choices at this point is always a good thing but breaking your diet a little bit isn't going to kill you. As I said above, if you want those greasy french fries, or that dessert after dinner, go for it. Just don't order two entrees, three desserts, eat the entire loaf of bread with butter and half of your spouse's dinner and then hit the ice cream place on the way home, call it a 'meal', and think I somehow gave you permission to do so.

Guidelines for the free meal

There aren't any real guidelines for the free meal beyond what I wrote above: don't use the concept as an excuse to eat yourself sick or eat three times what you'd normally eat. Just go eat a non-diet meal that lets you eat some of the off limits stuff and that's it. I do, however, want to give you some suggestions on the free meal.

Under most circumstances, I think a free meal is best eaten out of the house, at a restaurant. This is because you're less likely to go nuts on your total food intake at a restaurant (unless you go to an all you can eat buffet type of place which I don't suggest). You won't order three desserts (unless you want funny looks from the wait staff and your friends) or eat three meals, which is a real possibility if you eat this meal at home. Also, the going out aspect of the meal gives it more of a reward type of flavor, a special treat for your dieting efforts.

I also think it's best to make the free meal a dinner meal. The reason for this suggestion has to do with getting back into the swing of the diet. If you make your free meal lunch or breakfast, it can be psychologically difficult to go back to your diet for the rest of the day. If you make dinner your free meal, by the time you wake up in the morning, you should be ready to get back into your normal dieting rhythm. If you're on an exercise program, especially if you're doing weight training, it would be ideal to put the free meal on a day when you exercised.

As above, it would probably be ideal if you at least kept up some of the parameters of your normal diet and make relatively healthy choices. Just go ahead and have some of the forbidden stuff too. So try to make sure and get a source of protein and a salad at least, something healthy. To that you can add some of the forbidden stuff. The low-carber might add a baked potato or some bread (or dessert), the low-fat dieter might add fries or something greasy, as I mentioned above.

Some previous approaches to the free meal concept (for example Protein Power by the Eades) have further limited the free meal to one hour in duration. This may be helpful if it keeps you from turning what should be one meal into a several hour graze (and then rationalizing that it was only one 'meal'). At the same time, don't fall into the trap of seeing how much food you can eat in an hour if you do this. I've known of folks who literally start a stopwatch and see how much they can cram down their throat in an exact one-hour span (these same types of people often take it further during structured refeeds, described in the next chapter). Then they wonder why they aren't losing fat and bitch at me because they can't follow directions.

I want to give you one final warning: do not be surprised if your body weight spikes a little bit the next morning, especially if you eat a lot of carbohydrates at your free meal (this is more true for folks on low-carbohydrate diets). Avoiding the scale the morning after a free meal may be a good idea, especially if you are the type of person who gets overly concerned about short-term spikes in body weight.

Frequency and timing of free meals

With few exceptions, I feel that all dieters, regardless of what category they are in should incorporate, 1 or 2 free meals per week into their diet. This includes bodybuilders getting ready for a contest although they may find that structured refeeds (discussed next chapter) are a little more appropriate. A good friend, David Greenwalt (author of the excellent book The Leanness Lifestyle) has prepared for bodybuilding contests, reaching 4-5% body fat while including free meals into his diet.

I will say that if you're just starting a new diet, I think it's probably best to be relatively strict with it (allowing no free meals) for the first few weeks, mainly to give yourself time to get into the swing of the new eating habits. Taste buds take time to adjust and adding free meals in too early can be a way to prevent you from getting away from the types of foods that made you fat in the first place. Quite in fact, people often find that several weeks of relatively strict dieting tend to eliminate the taste they had for certain types of foods (whatever isn't allowed on the diet) and they tend to go less crazy during free meals. But this takes a few weeks at least to occur.

At that point, the free meals can be incorporated. Finally, you should generally space out your free meals on nonconsecutive days, rather than having them on two days in a row. So rather than having a free meal on Thursday and again on Friday, have one on Wednesday night and the other on Saturday (perhaps as part of some type of social event or special occasion). Oh yeah, don't try to be cute and have a free meal on Saturday, Sunday, Monday and Tuesday and try to rationalize that you only had 2 each week. Space them out on nonconsecutive days, you are still on a diet.

Structured refeeds Part 1

The next 'level' up from free meals are structured refeeds which are deliberate periods of high-carbohydrate overfeeding that may last anywhere from 5 hours (at the shortest) to one day (12-24 hours, probably the average) up to three days (for example, in my Ultimate Diet 2.0 book). Although a structured refeed has psychological benefits similar to the free meals, it has additional physiological benefits that the free meal lacks. To avoid a monstrous chapter length, I'm going to divide the discussion of refeeds into two sections and discuss some general ideas in this chapter and details in the next chapter.

I want to say right away that the structured refeed should be high-carbohydrate (and ideally fairly low in fat) regardless of the type of diet you are currently following. So whether you are on a high-carb/low-fat diet to begin with, living in The Zone, or doing a low-carbohydrate diet such as Atkins or The South Beach Diet or what have you, structured refeeds are a time to jack up the carbohydrates and lower your fat intake. I'll mention this repeatedly but this means that folks on moderate or higher fat diets will need to make a conscious effort to lower their habitual fat intake if they do a structured refeed.

I should also mention that a structured refeed would take the place of a free meal. So if your current diet was set up to include 2 free meals per week and you were doing a structured refeed for 5 hours once per week, you'd only get one free meal and one refeed that week. You do not get to add them together and do 2 free meals and the refeed.

I also want to point out upfront that even more than the free meal, structured refeeds have a real tendency to spike body weight because of the increased storage of carbohydrate in muscles and liver. Every gram of carbohydrate stored stores an addition 3 grams of water and this can add up to a rather considerable amount when a lot of carbs are eaten.

If you live and die by the scale, I'd really recommend not weighing for a few days after a structured refeed. If you do, don't freak out over the scale weight going up, it's just water weight which will drop back off soon enough. Unless you really screw up with the types of foods that you're eating (see below), you aren't putting on body fat.

Physiological benefits of the structured refeed

Beyond the potential psychological benefits of just letting eat all of the high-carbohydrate goodies that you're probably craving, structured refeeds have additional physiological benefits I want to mention first before I get into the details.

One of these is the refilling of muscle glycogen (carbohydrate stored within the muscle) which is important for individuals involved in high-intensity exercise such as weight training. Tangentially: depletion of muscle glycogen is often used as an argument against low-carbohydrate diets for folks who are doing intensive exercise. However, there are dietary approaches which alternate periods of low-carbohydrate dieting with high-carbohydrate consumption (usually called cyclical ketogenic diets or CKD's, discussed in detail in my first book, The Ketogenic Diet) are often used by athletes to combine low-carbohydrate dieting (which is extremely effective for some but not all dieters) while still allowing them to sustain their exercise regimens.

Structured refeeds achieve this goal as well. Many people (again, some but not all; I don't want you to read these comments as necessarily pro-low carbohydrate) seem to need to almost nearly eliminate carbohydrates from their diet to control their food intake, incorporating refeeds allows them to do this and perform intensive exercise.

Structured refeeds also temporarily turn off diet induced catabolism (roughly: tissue breakdown), helping to spare LBM/muscle loss. This becomes more and more important as people get leaner (into dieting Category 1) and is more important for people who are exercising than those who are not. Done properly, structured refeeds can be used to rebuild muscle that is often lost on a diet. This is discussed in more detail in my Ultimate Diet 2.0 which is aimed at individuals who are already in Category 1 and want to get extremely lean while maintaining (or increasing) both muscle mass and strength or performance.

Finally, and perhaps most importantly relative to most readers of this booklet, deliberately overeating carbohydrates helps to normalize most, if not all, of the hormones I talked about back in the chapter about body weight regulation: leptin, ghrelin, insulin, peptide YY, etc. Overeating carbohydrates works to normalize all of these hormones. I want to mention that overeating the other nutrients (fats and proteins) doesn't have the same effects on all of these hormones which is why structured refeeds need to be high-carbohydrate (and as I'll mention again below, low in fat) regardless of the type of diet that you're on. So whereas free meals is really just a time to eat whatever foods your current diet doesn't allow (if you want), refeeds should be high carbs and low fat for all dieters.

I should mention that it is somewhat debatable whether short refeeds (1 day or less) have much of an impact on metabolic rate, appetite or hormone levels. A recent study (in rats, unfortunately) found a short period of overfeeding in rats did increase metabolic rate but it's unknown if this applies to humans. Even if a structured refeed doesn't significantly

42

impact on metabolic rate, it serves the other purposes I mentioned: allowing a psychological break from dieting, refilling muscle glycogen and briefly turning of diet induced catabolism.

But first, the obligatory warning and comments on what not to do

Just as with the free meals, there are a couple of rather standard abuse patterns that people tend to fall into when they start doing refeeds (or cheat days as some sources call them). I'd say that the main one is going out of their way to see just how much food they can stuff down their pie hole in whatever time period they have been allotted (I'll talk about durations of refeeds in the next chapter).

Along with that, people have a tendency to interpret "Overeat carbohydrates for 12-24 hours" as "Eat nothing but junk food for 12-24 hours straight." I've heard of people who are doing a cheat day literally setting an alarm for 12:01 am and eating nothing but the worst crap they can find until 11:59 the next night, to ensure that they get exactly their 24 hours of cheating in. Then they wonder why their diet isn't working. Clearly, this is an abuse of what I'm talking about.

Along with that is the same pattern with the free meal but on a larger scale: they seem to go out of their way to put the worst kind of crap foods down their gullet during a refeed. This is important because, while I don't have a problem with certain kinds of junk foods (mainly the high-carb, low fat type stuff that people have been overconsuming for the last few years, think Snackwells cookies or low-fat ice cream or yogurt and stuff), I find a lot of people gorging on a lot of high carb and high-fat stuff (think donuts, cookies, full fat ice cream) and that causes a lot of problems.

Keep in mind that the goal of the structured refeed is to eat a lot of carbohydrates, not a lot of carbohydrates and fat. There are plenty enough high-carbohydrate, low-fat types of foods out there to keep most people happy. Many people, once they've lost their taste for high-sugar foods will just do refeeds with a lot of starches, bagels, bread, pasta and the like and ignore the junkier stuff; most seem to prefer a mixture. I'll talk more about types of foods in a second.

Along with that, people throw out all sense of decent nutrition that they have developed on whatever diet they are currently following. They go from following what it, hopefully, a sane diet and eat the worst crap they can. As with the free meal, I'd like to see folks getting at least some good nutrition during a refeed, which means lean proteins and some vegetables or fruits during their refeed. To that, they can add some of the high-carbohydrate goodies that are currently forbidden on their diet. That's a much better approach overall than going with the all junk food refeed.

Some general guidelines for the structured refeed

I mentioned some of the common problems that occur with refeeds above in the warning and I want to reiterate that structured refeeds should not be used as an excuse or rationale to see how much crappy food you can stuff down your gullet. Rather, we are trying to use foods (in this case, carbohydrates) to cause specific effects related to the physiological response to dieting.

This is part of why I've avoided calling it a cheat day in this booklet (as I have called it in the past and many continue to call it), people tend to think of 'cheating' as not only something that is negative but something that should be negative. So they fall out of one negative trap right into another.

So let's not think of this as a cheat day, let's fancy it up a bit. Rather, is it a structured refeed to affect specific physiological processes in the body. Barry Sears wasn't wrong when he said that eating is a hormonal event and, in this case, by eating a lot of carbohydrates over a specific period of time, we're causing specific hormonal processes to be affected.

That is to say a little less convolutedly, the goal of a structured refeed is not simply to overeat carbohydrates for the sake of overeating carbohydrates (although that alone may provide some psychological benefit) but to do so for specific physiological reasons: normalizing the hormones which are regulating body weight, refilling muscle glycogen, etc. Hopefully conceptualizing it that way will prevent you from going out of control and falling into the traps I described above.

First things first, no matter how you do a refeed, I really want to emphasize that you need to get sufficient amounts of lean proteins (think chicken, fish, lean red meats, low or nonfat dairy) and some veggies or fruits (both for their nutritional value and for their fiber) with your high carbohydrate intake. And while fat intake should be kept low (see below), if you're worrying about the essential fatty acids (such as flax oil or fish oils), make sure to get those too. This not only ensures that you meet good basic nutritional requirements but the inclusion of protein, fiber and a small amount of dietary fat with every high carbohydrate meal will keep blood sugar more stable and make you feel a lot better.

I want to really emphasize again the need to keep dietary fat intake fairly low while doing a structured refeed, 50 grams of fat (about 4 tablespoons) should be about the maximum (note: 50 grams will seem high to people on a low-carbohydrate diet, normal to folks in the Zone and low to people on most popular low-carbohydrate diets). And I do suggest that you track/measure your fat intake (translation: read labels, get out the measuring spoon) because it's extremely easy to overeat fat if you're not careful.

This means that people on a low-carb/high-fat type of diet will need to lower their fat intake significantly when they do a refeed. So if you're used to eating fatty meat and full fat cheese and such on a low-carbohydrate diet, you really need to make sure and cut the fat intake down significantly by making different food choices. I can't emphasize this enough, a combination of a lot of carbohydrates and fat is a wonderful way to regain body fat during a structured refeed; if you're going to jack up carbohydrates, you must cut back your dietary fat intake.

Again, I want to mention that the refeed takes the place of a free meal. So if you're currently taking two free meals per week and decide to incorporate a structured refeed, you would only get one free meal and the refeed that week. Category 1 dieters who are doing 2 short refeeds per week (see next chapter) would take no free meals, only the refeeds. Basically, don't try to push the limits of your diet by trying to add refeeds to the free meals.

Types of carbohydrates: Some general comments

So let's talk about types of carbohydrates; I'll deal with amounts in the next chapter. For the most part, I like to see structured refeeds centered around dietary starches such as breads, bagels, pasta, rice, potatoes, etc. All of those foods that the low-carbohydrate diet books say are bad for you.

Some junk food is ok (and probably desirable) but too much sucrose (table sugar) or fructose (fruit sugar) tends to cause problems relating to fat regain. I should mention that the fructose content of fruit really isn't a huge problem; rather, high fructose corn syrup, found in almost any refined carbohydrate food you see on the grocery store shelf contributes the excessive fructose intakes that are causing problems in our modern world. You can have some sucrose and fructose, it just shouldn't be the totality of your refeed.

100 grams of sucrose (this is easy to go over if you eat a lot of candy or junk food) and 50 grams of fructose (which is a probably 5-7 normal pieces of fruit or a rather small amount of most refined foods) should be about the maximum during a refeed and this does limit the types of foods you can eat somewhat.

So all starches, moderate amounts of fruit (2-3 pieces total), and even some junk food (again, not too much) is fair game. This should give you plenty of food freedom and allow you to fulfill any nagging carbohydrate cravings (people tend to crave carbs more than anything else on a diet) without causing problems.

So you might focus on breads, pasta, bagels, potatoes, rice and foods of that nature for your starches. A few pieces of fruit and a bit of junky food (think nonfat ice cream or sherbet, Snackwell's types of cookies, candy like jelly beans or candy corns or some such) can round out your total intake.

Finally, I want to mention that some people simply do not feel good when they do structured refeeds; this tends to be especially true of those folks who feel the best on low-carbohydrate diets. This is commonly true with individuals suffering from some degree of insulin resistance (roughly: their bodies don't respond well to the hormone insulin). They get major blood sugar swings (highs and lows) which can cause some pretty large scale energy swings. Most people feel crappy when their blood glucose crashes (this also tends to stimulate hunger) and refeeds can cause that.

Getting adequate protein, fiber and a small amount of dietary fat with each high-carbohydrate meal goes a long way towards solving this problem. If adding those to your high-carbohydrate intake doesn't solve the problem (this is especially true for Category 3 dieters and to a lesser degree everyone else), you have basically two options. The first is to pick much more unrefined carbohydrate sources, whole grains and such and avoid all of

45

the refined stuff. Alternately, it may simply be that refeeds aren't a good idea at this point and you should stick with free meals and full diet breaks for the time being. I'll mention this again in the next chapter.

Structured Refeeds Part 2

In the last chapter, I made some general comments about structured refeeds, including the obligatory warning about what not to do. As well, I made a few basic comments about the purpose of the refeeds (both psychological and physiological) and addressed some of the issues surrounding food choices. In this chapter, I want to get into the details of how often and for how long (duration and frequency) dieters should perform a structured refeed.

The structured refeed: Duration

So how does one do a structured refeed? Unlike the free meal which is fairly simple, when looking at the structured refeed we have to look at three different components: the duration of the refeed, the frequency of refeeds and the types/amounts of foods that should be consumed. I made some general comments about food types in the last chapter and here I want to focus on the duration and frequency of the refeeds.

To make it a bit simpler (I've fought with the structure of this chapter for weeks now), I'm going to describe three different length refeeds which are 5 hours, 1 day and 2 days. For details on a longer refeed like the 3 days of the Ultimate Diet 2.0, you'll just have to buy that book (sorry, I have bills to pay, too). The duration of each refeed along with a range of carbohydrate intakes appears in table 1 below.

Table 1: Amount of carbohydrate for different length refeeds

Length of refeed	Amount of carbohydrate
5 hours	1.5-3 grams/pound LBM (~3-6 g/kg)
1 day	4-6 g/lb LBM (~8-12 g/kg)
2 days	2-3 g/lb (~4-6 g/kg)

Note: Obviously you'll have to do a bit of math, multiplying the above values by your lean body mass (estimated back in Chapter 8) to determine how many carbs to eat. As a general rule, individuals in exercise Category 1 would use the higher values and individuals in exercise Category 2 would use the lower values. As I'll mention below, all dieters may benefit from starting at the low end of the range and seeing how they respond. If well, they can increase the amount of carbohydrates eaten at subsequent refeeds.

General comments on the above: timing and scheduling

Before giving frequency recommendations, I want to make some comments about the refeed durations listed above. 5 hours should be pretty clear, it means that the refeed will last 5 hours total from start to finish. So from 4pm to 9pm or 5 pm to 10 pm for example.

1 day means morning to night but remember my warnings from the last chapter: this really means from breakfast until dinner, don't fall into the trap of waking up at 12:01am and seeing how much food you can eat until 11:59pm the next evening.

2 days means morning to evening for 2 consecutive days. While previous approaches (such as Bodyopus) required that dieters wake up in the middle of the night to eat, this tends to be beyond what most people are willing to do (obsessive athletes excepted). It's generally sufficient to simply end the first day's refeed with a large carbohydrate meal at bedtime and then start again at breakfast the next morning.

Ideally, the total carbohydrate intake of the structured refeed should be spread across the entire time frame, with a meal occurring every 2-3 hours or so. This is important to keep blood glucose and insulin up/stable which both avoids problems with energy crashes and helps to upregulate all of the hormonal systems that we are addressing. Eating all of your food in one sitting is simply ineffective. As with the free meal, I suggest that you end the refeed at bedtime which means you'll have to count backwards for however many hours the refeed is planned to last.

So let's say you've got a 5 hour refeed scheduled and typically go to bed at 9pm. 9pm would be your last meal and 4 pm would be your first so you'd, ideally, put another meal about halfway between or around 6:30pm. A 1 day refeed would run from morning to bedtime so you would start the refeed at, say, 9am and eat every 3 hours or so until bedtime at 9pm. So that would be 9am, 12pm, 3pm, 6pm and 9pm. That would be ideal anyway. Clearly if your work or daily schedule won't allow that ideal structure, you'll simply have to do the best that you can. One solution is to refeed on the weekends (which may have other benefits I'll mention below). If you must refeed during a work day, snacks between major meals may be the best way to get in your carbohydrate allotment.

For a 2 day refeed, you'd go from breakfast until dinner on day 1. You would ideally finish with a large carbohydrate meal at bedtime (this will continue digesting during some portion of the night) and then get up the next morning and continue. If you happened to wake up in the middle of the night (to use the bathroom, for example), you could eat some more carbohydrates as part of a 2 day refeed but I don't think forcing yourself to get up every few hours is useful or necessary under most conditions.

For exercisers, it would be ideal to synchronize an exercise sessions (preferably weight training) with the refeed. For a 5 hour refeed, a large carbohydrate meal about an hour prior to workout followed by a big carb meal right after the workout and again 2 hours later would be just about perfect. For the longer refeeds, if you can work out first thing in the morning, that's probably ideal. If not, simply try to get a workout in sometime during that day. And, well, if you're not currently exercising, either consider starting or just don't worry about it.

Clearly, because of their length, the suggestion (as per the free meal) to eat out is unrealistic for a structured refeed That means that a bit more self-control will be necessary to keep your food intake under control. What some dieters have done with good success is not go shopping until they are about to do the refeed which avoids problems with keeping those types of diet breaker foods in the house. As well, some dieters only buy what they intend to eat for a given refeed which avoids the problems of vastly overconsuming carbohydrates if things get out of control. So if they are supposed to eat, say 500 grams of carbohydrates during their free meal, they'll buy exactly that many and that's what they'll eat during the refeed. Yes, this does require you to read food labels.

As with the free meal, it's generally best to try and end the refeed at bedtime, to make it easier to return to your diet the next morning. This really only applies to the 5 hour refeed anyhow but trying to refeed from 8am until 1pm and then go back to dieting for the rest of the day tends to be difficult for most people. The 1 and 2 day refeeds start at breakfast and end at dinnertime by definition.

As a final comment, which I think I've alluded to already, some people find that they get rather major energy swings during refeeds, even if they follow all of my guidelines. There are a number of physiological reasons for this which aren't that relevant; sufficed to say that this happens. For this reason, you may wish to schedule a refeed on a day when you're not working, so that you're not dealing with the fatigue that can accompany wide blood sugar swings. That would be Saturday or Sunday for most people. Refeeds can also be structured around special events or just generally around the weekends since that's when most people want to go out, be sociable and such.

Structured refeeds: Frequency

Now that you have information about the different durations of the structured refeeds and how many carbohydrates to consume it's time to address frequency. In this regards, free meals were far easier, everyone got one or two free meals per week. Refeeds are more complicated.

A lot of the choice of how often and how long to refeed depends on factors such as how hard you're dieting (the harder you're dieting, the more often you need to refeed), starting body fat percentage (taken into account below), activity patterns (people involved in more high intensity exercise need more frequent and generally longer refeeds) and others that are simply impossible to describe in a book format and give guidelines for.

The recommendations I'm going to present below are sort of average recommendations based on a mix of science, experimentation, experience, intuition and just a bit of guesswork. They represent average recommendations and nothing more and readers may have to play around a bit with refeeds to find what works best.   If you're really completely lost on the structured refeed concept, just drop me an email or something (check the front of the book) and I'll do my best to help. Or just skip it entirely and stick with free meals and the full diet break discussed next chapter.

As a general rule, as with amounts, the best choice for all dieters is to start with the shorter duration refeeds to see how they respond. If the response is good, they don't have problems returning to their previous diet, they don't seem to regain a bunch of weight that doesn't come back off (which would suggest a true fat regain) and their diet proceeds better after the refeed, they can increase the time towards the longer durations. If the response is poor and no major mistakes (in terms of amounts or types of foods) were made, it may indicate that the dieter shouldn't do refeeds (I'll come back to this below).

Recall from a few chapters back that the exercise categories are as follows: Category 1 is for individuals involved in fairly intensive weight training 2-3 days per week for at least an hour, or long duration or high intensity endurance exercise and Category 2 is for everyone else. That means that Category 2 includes people who are not exercising, people only doing low to moderate intensity aerobic exercise, or people just lifting baby weights in the gym who don't work very hard.

Table 2: Frequency and duration of refeeds				
Diet category		Exercise category	Duration	Frequency
1		1	5 hours-1 day	Every 3 to 5 days
	OR	1	1-2 days	Every 7 days
1		2	1 day	Every 7-10 days
2		1	5 hours	Every 7 days
2	OR	1	1 day	10-14 days
		2	5 hours-1 days	Every 14 days
3		1	5 hours	Every 10-14 days
3		2	5 hours-1 day	Every 21 days

50

You may notice above that refeeds become longer and more frequent as dieters get leaner which may seem counterintuitive. The basic reason is that the physiological issues related to dieting in terms of metabolic slowdown and the rest tend to become more pronounced as people get leaner and leaner. For someone not genetically disposed to it, trying to get below 10% body fat is essentially no different than starving to death (from the body's perspective): keeping things moving means refeeding more frequently.

As well, the exercise category that a dieter is in determines a great deal of how often to refeed occurs and how long it should be. For the most part, that is the major distinction I'm making above in terms of how often and how long to do a refeed for; exercise Category 1 people need to refeed more often and for longer than exercise Category 2 people.

This has to do with the effect of exercise on muscle glycogen stores, intensive (or extremely long duration, I'm talking several hours here) exercise depleting muscle glycogen. This means that refeeds need to be performed more often if for no other reason than to refill muscle glycogen and help to sustain exercise performance while dieting.

Category 1 dieters

In general, Category 1 dieters are athletes and bodybuilder types who are trying to get extra lean for either competition or appearance reasons. Meaning they are generally in exercise Category 1, involved in fairly intensive weight and/or endurance training. Which isn't to say that there couldn't be non-athlete individuals in this Category, I simply doubt they are in the majority.

Unless they are genetically predisposed towards staying lean (in which case they probably aren't reading this booklet), Category 1 dieters tend to have the worst problems with metabolic slowdown and the rest of the issues I described back in Chapter 3 which is the main reason that I suggest that they do a refeed as often and for as long as I do. Psychological stuff is a little less predictable, usually folks at that level are pretty good about their diets and aren't trying to fix long-standing food control issues. At the same time, dieting to extreme leanness is usually a miserable experience and the psychological benefits of free meals and refeeds are important as well.

As I mentioned already, Category 1 dieters tend to be involved in either a lot (endurance athletes) or fairly high intensity (everybody else) activity. This means that they tend to deplete a lot of glycogen and exercise performance can become a very real issue along with everything else. Frankly, Category 1 dieters would probably be better off with something like my Ultimate Diet 2.0 (you're probably wondering just how many times I can mention that damn thing) but not everybody wants a plan that rigid or extreme which is why I'm discussing general flexible dieting approaches here.

Because of the amount of glycogen depleting exercise that they do, overall good muscular insulin sensitivity and everything else, individuals in this category who are in exercise Category 1 can 'get away' with the most during their structured refeeds. This includes both the amount of carbs that they can consume as well as the types; Category 1 dieters can consume the largest amounts of carbs and tend to handle junkier stuff a little bit better.

Which isn't to say that most can get away with all junk-food refeeds, simply that there tends to be more leeway.

I want to note here that the only difference between exercise Category 1 and 2 dieters is that Category 2 dieters should always start with the lower amount of carbohydrate recommendations; since they aren't as glycogen depleted going into the refeed, excess carbohydrates tend to have more problems 'spilling over' into fat cells. With that said, let's look at amounts of carbohydrates for each of the different length refeeds.

As per table 1, for 5 hour refeeds, a range of 1.5-3 grams of carbohydrate per pound of lean body mass (roughly 3-6.5 grams/kg for metrically inclined readers) is suggested. So for someone with 160 pounds of lean body mass, that's 240-480 grams of carbohydrates over a 5 hour span which would be divided up roughly evenly across 3 meals. That's 80-160 grams of carbs per meal. Which really isn't that much when you start looking at some of the more highly concentrated starches (some of the bigger bagels can contain 40 grams of carbs, for example and a big bowl of pasta probably contains that many carbohydrates easily).

As well, depending on the level of glycogen depletion, some people can get away with far more carbohydrates than that. Again, I strongly suggest starting conservatively and increasing the amounts based on your results. If you find yourself getting fuller (muscularly) and leaner after your refeeds, you can try increasing the amounts. If you find yourself waking up flat and puffy, you either ate too many total carbohydrates or ate too much sucrose or fructose and need to alter either the quality or quantity of your refeed.

For longer refeeds, the amounts of carbs that can and should be consumed go up as you would expect. For a 1 day refeed, somewhere between 4-6 grams/pound of lean body mass (about 9-13 grams/kilogram) is going to be appropriate. So our 160 pound lean body mass individual would consume somewhere between 640 and 960 grams of carbohydrates over this time span. Over 6 or so meals, you're looking at somewhere between 100 and 160 grams per meal or so.

If you work it out, eating this amount of carbohydrates along with protein and moderate amounts of fat will tend to raise calories to maintenance or higher levels. If you're wondering why the numbers are slightly different than what I presented in my Ultimate diet 2.0, it's because I can't be sure that Category 1 dieters are completely glycogen depleted going into the refeed; hence I'm erring on the side of too few carbs rather than too many.

The reason that you don't just get fat again is that, in the short-term, incoming carbohydrates go to muscle and liver glycogen first, energy production second, and fat storage last. So under conditions of glycogen depletion, the body can handle this type of calorie overload in the short-term without getting fat. The issue of calorie partitioning is discussed in excruciating detail in, you guessed it, The Ultimate Diet 2.0.

Finally, for a 2 day refeed, dieters simply add a second day of carbohydrate overfeeding to the standard 1 day refeed. Since muscle glycogen stores will have been replenished greatly, you don't get to eat nearly as many carbohydrates or calories during the second day of refeeding. So while 4-6 grams/lb was appropriate for the first 24 hours, perhaps half of that or an additional 2-3 grams/lb (4-6 grams/kg or so) would be appropriate during the second 24 hours.

Category 2

Category 2 dieters are probably the most difficult to pin down. They may be athletes who have gotten out of shape (or are in a sport where being a lard-ass doesn't hurt them that much) or non-athletes who simply want to lose a little bit of body fat/weight for appearance or some other reason. Physiologically, they are basically in-between Category 1 and 3 in terms of metabolic issue, hunger control, insulin sensitivity and the rest. Psychologically, they might have decent food control but have gotten a bit sloppy, or they may just be a bit overweight and be trying to overhaul their eating completely. Basically, I can't make tremendous predictions on what's going on in this category.

For individuals in exercise Category 1 (performing regular, fairly intensive weight training), the recommendations above are either a 5 hour refeed once a week or a full day refeeding every 10-14 days. I should note that a Category 2 dieter who is involved in large amounts of intensive activity may need to move to the refeed recommendations for Category 1 dieters. That is, if they are depleting their muscle glycogen on a nearly weekly basis, they will need to do a refeed more often.

Individuals in exercise Category 2 are far easier to make recommendations for. General daily activity will gradually deplete muscle glycogen but not very rapidly. As well, the generally decreased problem with metabolic slowdown and the rest means that a refeed isn't necessary all that often. A 5 hour to 1 day refeed every 2 weeks should generally be sufficient. Once again, I suggest that dieters start with the lower end of the range (both in terms of duration and carbohydrate amount) to assess their response and then increase both as long as that response is positive.

Category 3

It's debatable whether Category 3 dieters really *need* a refeed as part of their overall diet structure although the reasons are more complicated than I want to get into in this booklet. Just note that they probably aren't really required in the same way as for the Category 1 and 2 dieters; I'm including them as an option for completeness.

Category 3 dieters are often dealing with some rather long-standing food control issues which refeeds have the potential to derail. It's too easy, just into a new diet to let a refeed put them right back into the eating habits they are trying to fix. This is especially true if they don't heed my warning regarding the pitfalls to avoid from the last chapter.

As I mentioned before, taste buds take time (3-6 weeks) to adapt to a new style of eating and habits take time to become entrenched. Most psychologists will tell you that it takes at least 3 weeks to establish a new pattern and I find it no coincidence that most people drop out of new diet and exercise programs about the 3 week mark, just before it's starting to become a habit.

As well, Category 3 people are often insulin resistant (roughly: their bodies don't respond well to the hormone insulin) in the first place and high-carbohydrate eating as necessitated by the structured refeed can often cause the very problems that they are trying to avoid. For these reasons, Category 3 dieters may wish to forego structured refeeds (despite their appeal) for the first 5-6 weeks or so of their new diet.

Waiting 5-6 weeks will give them time to adjust to the new eating habits and the weight loss will improve insulin sensitivity. A short (5 hour) refeed can then be attempted to see what the response is. As mentioned above, if a Category 3 dieter finds that a structured refeed does more harm than good, making it hard for them to get back on their diet afterwards or what have you, they should be discontinued.

Alternately, Category 3 dieters may want to avoid refeeds completely and only include free meals and full diet breaks (see next chapter) initially. Once they move into dieting Category 2, including structured refeeds will become more necessary and should be incorporated as suggested above.

A few final comments on refeeds and an alternative method to scheduling

As I mentioned, the above guidelines for frequency, duration, and amounts of carbohydrates are based on about one-half research, one-half experience, one-half intuition and one-half guesswork. Yes, I know that adds to more than one.

Anyhow, I have found that the above guidelines work fairly well for a majority of people. But there are always outliers when you deal with human biology and I want to mention a few exceptions to the above.

First are folks who diet just fine without refeeds. They are in a small minority but they are there; I suspect they are part of that spendthrift metabolic type I mentioned elsewhere. Invariably these folks don't see the reason or rationale for refeeds but are seemingly unaware that they are, metabolically speaking, in the minority. Since they don't seem to need them, they can't see why anybody else would.

As well, some people seem to respond staggeringly poorly to refeeding, especially if it's done for too long or too frequently. They tend to report extreme weight gains that just doesn't come back off as it should and the refeeds end up hurting their diet more than helping it. Frankly, I don't know why this is the case exactly but I've seen it often enough to know that it occurs. If you find that you are in this category, and you're not screwing up in terms of amounts of carbs or your food choices choices, you should probably stick with just the free meals and full diet breaks (described next chapter).

By the same token, there will be people for whom the above average frequency/duration recommendations don't seem to pan out exactly; they are close but not quite right. For this reason I want to describe an alternative method to scheduling refeeds although I want to preface this with a warning that it is very easy to screw up.

This method, basically a subjective approach to refeeding, is premised on the fact that you are in pretty good tune with your own body (and mind) and can be extremely honest with yourself. It becomes far too easy to rationalize refeeds altogether too frequently with what I'm about to describe. If you think you might be in this category, you may want to just skip to the next chapter, what I'm going to describe is just going to give you dangerous ideas.

Back in chapter 3 I talked little bit about some of the adaptations that occur with dieting in terms of metabolic rate slowdown and the rest. One of the adaptations I described was an increase in hunger/appetite. I should have actually made a distinction between the two in that chapter but it wasn't really that important; so I'm making it now.

In scientific terms hunger refers to a short-term desire for food. So you get hungry, you eat a meal, you get full, you stop eating. Appetite describes a longer term drive for food. Clearly, they overlap. An example that may help make this more clear is that older individuals frequently report a drop in overall appetite but they still get hungry. So they'll still get hungry, eat a meal, get full and stop; but their overall food intake is decreased. The brain chemistry controlling these different systems is complicated to say the least.

One of the key molecules in all of this, though, is a compound called neuropeptide Y or NPY. When NPY levels go up in the brain, the body's entire attention seems to be drawn to food. Quite in fact, rats injected with NPY will forego sex for sugar water. Basically, it's yet another biological process trying to keep you alive, when you're starving to death (and dieting is just starvation on a lesser scale), eventually your body makes you think about nothing about food. I should mention that NPY (along with a host of other brain chemicals) is also involved in the metabolic rate slowdown, hormonal problems, and all the rest I described in a previous chapter.

I'm bringing this up because dieters (especially as they get leaner) tend to reach a point where they move beyond just being hungry. They find that they are basically obsessed with food. Often, and this is where being in good touch with their bodies is key, they can almost feel the various biological systems (metabolic rate, etc.) shutting down. Energy drops, they feel lethargic, sex drives goes down, etc.; they can just feel it happening. Yeah, I know, this sounds flaky and new agey but it does happen to some people. And it's a very good indication that NPY levels are off the scale and that a refeed should be performed.

This, more so than arbitrary guidelines, is a good signal that a structured refeed (or full diet break, see next chapter) is necessary. And it's one way to program structured refeeds into your overall diet. Again, I offer it as an alternative but only if you can really be honest with yourself and have a very good feeling of what your body is telling you. You need a good ability to differentiate basic diet induced hunger from the type of all consuming obsession with food that occurs when NPY levels really skyrocket. As above, it becomes all too easy to decide, altogether too frequently that you really 'need' a structured refeed. Then when you start wondering why your diet isn't working, well....

The Full Diet Break

Introduction

The next several chapters deal with two slightly different but still related concepts. If you read The Rapid Fat Loss Handbook, you will recognize them as essentially the same sets of information with slight modifications since the primary topic of the books are different.

Those two concepts are the full diet break mentioned back in Chapter 8 and the issue of moving to maintenance after your diet is over. As mentioned above, these are intimately related with the only real difference being one of duration. A full diet break is a short term approach, generally 14 days while maintenance eating is long-term, essentially maintaining good eating habits forever. So whenever I talk about doing a full diet break below, you can assume that the same applies to a dieter moving into maintenance eating when their diet is over. When there are differences between the two, I'll make note of it.

Before I cover anything else, I want to mention that it is not uncommon for body weight to spike by a few pounds when performing a full diet break. This is especially true for low-carbohydrate dieters who reintroduce carbs but can also occur in individual on moderate carb (Zone-type) or high-carb diets. This slight increase in no cause for alarm and represents increased glycogen (carbohydrate stored in the muscle) and water storage. As well, increased food in the gut can increase body weight slightly.

I also want to mention that when I originally wrote these chapters (the next four), it was easier to target them as everyone was coming off of the same diet (the one described in my Rapid Fat Loss Handbook). With this booklet, in that I'm not describing any specific singular dietary approach, I can't know for sure what diet readers are using. Someone coming off of a low-carb diet may need to do something slightly different than someone on a Zone or high-carb diet. So don't be surprised if some of my guidelines are a little bit vague at points. I will try to address specific diets when possible in the subsequent chapters.

Planned versus unplanned diet breaks

As mentioned in the foreword and throughout this book, situations invariably arise that make sticking to a diet basically impossible. It might be a vacation or the holidays or just a period when life becomes too hectic to stick to your diet. I'm going to refer to this, logically, enough as an unplanned diet break.

For example, a member of my forum had a situation where he was going snowboarding for 10 days, while in the middle of the diet described in my Rapid Fat Loss Handbook. He wanted to know how to maintain the diet during his vacation and we all told him that he shouldn't, that he should simply move to controlled eating patterns, do the best he can and not worry about dieting until afterwards. This is a perfect example of when a full diet break ends up being unplanned and I'm sure readers can think of many others.

As well, there are situations where I think dieters should deliberately go off of their diet for some time periods, and this is what I'm going call a planned diet break. Which raises the question of why someone who was having no real problems sticking to their diet would bother going off of it in the first place. I'll come back to this below when I talk about the purpose of a deliberate diet break.

Here I want to simply give my recommendations for how long you should diet prior to taking a planned diet break (this assumes that you don't have a situation of an unplanned diet break). As usual, the primary determination has to do with your body fat percentage, the leaner you get, the shorter period of time you should diet without taking a break. Table 1 sums up some average recommendations for how long to diet before taking a full diet break. Readers of my Rapid Fat Loss Handbook will notice that the numbers below are identical to the ones I gave in the last chapter of that booklet.

Dieting category and length of diet before a break	
Dieting category	Number of weeks on a diet before a break
1	4-6
2	6-12
3	12-16

As with the structured refeeds discussed last chapter, please realize that the above recommendations represent average values and some fluctuation can be expected. Some dieters, no matter how lean, find that they can diet for extended periods without any significant slowing of fat loss while others find that metabolism and the rest go haywire quickly. As always, take the above as a recommendation and estimation; it should not be interpreted as an immutable form of holy writ.

Controlled versus uncontrolled diet breaks

As far as I can tell, in the Wing study I cited a few chapters back, the dieting subjects were not given any recommendations on what or how to eat during their planned diet breaks. I'll only note that, whatever they did, they didn't regain much (if any) weight and appear not to have lost total food control. I already mentioned some of the reasons I think it worked out this way in that chapter so I won't rehash that again.

I bring this up because many people, when faced with a situation where they have to take a break, fall into that same pattern I've described in the chapters on free meals and refeeds, they go from one extreme (strict dieting) to the opposite (seeing how much crap they can stuff down their gullet). This is quite similar to how most people handle ending a diet. Figuring that the diet is now over, they return to their old (usually poor) eating habits and gain back all the weight and fat or maybe even a little bit more. Now I suppose if you don't really care about regaining a ton (or all) of weight or fat back during your full diet break (or after the diet is over), I certainly can't stop you. It's pretty safe to say that that's not my preferred method for engaging in a full diet break.

A sort of semi-controlled diet break would mean simply doing damage control, sort of following your overall current diet but not being too obsessive about it. Even if you ate 'properly' (where properly means whatever diet you're currently on) most of the day and had what amounted to a free meal every night, you'd still be way ahead of the game compared to the folks who are chowing down on nothing but crap food at every meal. This is obviously another option and one that some are capable of following. Once again, this type of approach takes a fundamental reworking of your attitude towards dieting. If you are the type of person who *only* follows a diet if you can be 100% and anything less than 100% means you are gorging on junk, well, maybe now you can see how damaging that can be. If you can get yourself into the mindset where doing your best is ok (at least in the short term), even when life won't allow perfection, you're primed to do much better in the long run.

But one premise of the past few (and the upcoming few chapters) is that not everybody can follow that sort of seat of the pants style of flexible dieting; some people need what amounts to a structured flexible dieting approach (as contradictory a concept as that is). So I'm going to give some guidelines in this and the upcoming chapters for how to approach a full diet break (or moving to maintenance after the diet is over) for people who want more control. As well, since I struggled for literally months to get these chapters written, I'm going to put them to use. You'll probably end up seeing them in the next few books I write in one form or another, just because they gave me such a headache.

The interaction of planned/unplanned and controlled/uncontrolled diet breaks

I suppose I should probably mention that whether the diet break is planned or unplanned may be a factor in whether or not it can be controlled or not. For example, consider my snowboarding forum member: odds are that he will not have staggering amounts of control over food availability as a consequence of being on vacation.

The same goes for almost any vacation or for the holidays when parties and other problematic situations arise constantly. Such situations tend not to lend themselves to high levels of dietary control although the information in the next two chapters can be put to some use to try and limit the damage. Of course, the most important facet (and the main premise of this book) is that eventually the situation forcing the unplanned diet break will end. By not losing long-term perspective, dieters can return to their diet, lose any weight that was gained, and get moving towards their goal again.

We might contrast this to someone who is taking a planned diet break as part of their overall plan. Odds are they will be in a far better situation to control their food intake as they probably aren't traveling or on holiday or vacation. The following chapters are probably of a bit more relevance to them although I encourage all readers to read them (especially the next two) as they deal with a information relevant to anyone trying to control their food or calorie intake.

What, exactly, is the purpose of the full diet break?

Before continuing, I want to go into a bit more detail of the goal of the full diet break, as this also gives me an easier segue into actually talking about it. In keeping with earlier chapters, and the rather artificial separation of psychology and physiology, a full diet break can fulfill both psychological and physiological needs.

The psychological ones should be fairly easy to understand: by breaking your dieting efforts up into smaller chunks, while maintaining control over your eating in the long-term, you are less likely to lose control or go off of your diet completely. This ties in with the basic premise of this entire book, that being more flexible about your eating habits, by gaining a better perspective about the realities of weight and fat loss, you are more likely to succeed in the long-run.

But what about physiological reasons? Even with the best diet and the proper use of free meals and structured refeeds, eventually the body adapts to a point where the diet that was once generating decent fat loss is no longer doing so. This adaptation is due to the systems I discussed in some detail a bunch of chapters back: it's an interaction of leptin and all of the other hormones which are telling the brain to adapt to fat loss by altering such metabolic processes as thyroid output and nervous system output (both of which have profound effects on metabolic rate).

By raising calories, we raise leptin (and normalize the other hormones) and metabolism tends to recover, helping the next phase of dieting work more effectively. Once again, of course, the goal is to try to fix metabolism without gaining back so much weight or fat that you end up worse off. Even then, let's say you gain a pound of real fat over the 2 week span of the full diet break. Compared to what you should have lost during the previous dieting phase, this is a drop in the bucket. As well, if that one or two pound gain means you lose fat at a faster rate when returning to your diet, it's more than worth it.

A quick diversion about metabolic rate slowdown

Although I discussed the different time courses for metabolic rate slowdown in the Rapid Fat Loss Handbook, I didn't do so that much in this book (my crafty way of making you buy both books). So I'm going to give you the abridged version here. In short, there are multiple reasons that metabolism slows on a diet, some of which are under our control and some of which aren't.

The factor that is mostly out of our control is the simple loss of body weight. A lighter body burns fewer calories at rest and during exercise and the loss of weight is one of the primary factors contributing to the reduction in daily caloric requirements. Clearly, short of regaining all of your lost weight, there's not much you can do about this. I did, however, mention one weird possibility (one that I'm surprised nobody else has really delved into), wearing a weighted vest or even a backpack with weight in it, to offset some of the weight loss. It wouldn't affect calorie burn at rest but you'd burn more calories during daily activity and this would probably help to offset some of the weight loss dependent reduction in caloric expenditure.

But there is an additional factor contributing to the metabolic rate slowdown, called the adaptive component. Basically, this represents a drop in caloric expenditure more than what you'd expect given the drop in body weight. Meaning this: let's say that we would predict metabolic rate to slow by 150 calories for a 10 pound weight loss. But when we actually measure the slowdown, the drop is 250 calories per day. The extra 100 calorie drop is the adaptive component.

What regulates the adaptive component? A lot of it is the changes in hormones that occur when you diet: leptin, insulin, thyroid, and nervous system output. One of the primary goals of the full diet break is to reset all of those hormones (to one degree or another) to try to correct the adaptive reduction in metabolic rate. This allows the diet to proceed more effectively when you reduce calories again.

The segue: The full diet break in brief

To achieve those goals, we need to accomplish two things during the full diet break. The first, and easiest is that dietary carbohydrate intake needs to be at least 100 grams per day. This is crucial for the upregulation of thyroid hormone which is one of the key players in regulating all of this. Raising leptin and insulin (and thus nervous system output) is also somewhat dependent on carbohydrate intake so you're going to have to raise your intake to at least that 100 g/day level.

That's the easy step although many low-carbohydrate dieters will freak out at the mere suggestion. People using a Zone type of diet or a high-carbohydrate diet are probably already consuming this many carbohydrates to begin with and won't need to worry about it so much. If you follow the recommendations I'm going to give for setting up a maintenance diet, you should get 100 grams of carbohydrates easily.

The second step, representing the segue into the next several chapters is that calories need to be raised to maintenance levels and I'll be referring to the full diet break as a maintenance diet from here on out (the name change is primarily to save me endless retyping of these chapters). Of course, the same exact information applies to moving to actual maintenance after a diet is over and some of what I'll talk about below applies more to long-term maintenance then the short-term diet break.

Defining a maintenance diet

So what is a maintenance diet? By definition, a maintenance diet is one that will maintain your current body weight or body fat level. Now, it would be unrealistic for you to maintain your body weight with zero fluctuations, changes in water balance and the rest will cause some fluctuations (women all know what can happen to their body weight during different parts of the menstrual cycle). The same goes for body fat levels although it usually takes longer term over- or undereating to cause body fat to change.

As well, nobody should expect themselves to eat an exactingly identical amount of food every day while doing an exacting amount of exercise. Ok, maybe obsessed bodybuilders but few without that particular psychology can be expected to do it in the long-term. In any event, that type of attitude goes against the whole premise of this booklet (and certainly of the full diet break) which is that being more relaxed about your diet is a better way to go in the long-term.

Let's be realistic: nobody is perfect every day of their life. More importantly, who wants to get to the end of their life, having had no enjoyment or pleasure, but being able to claim that their body weight never wavered even a bit? So let's relax our definition a bit and say that a maintenance diet (and exercise program) will maintain your body weight or body fat within a relatively narrow range, maybe 3-5 pounds either direction (with the big concern being an increase).

I should note that I would find that great a true fat gain during a full diet break to be extremely unusual. At worst, after the initial weight spike of a few pounds, you might gain a pound or two of fat if you really let your habits go to hell. Three to five pounds of true fat gain in a 2 week span would indicate some seriously bad eating habits. It can probably be done, mind you, especially over the holidays when you're surrounded by nothing but high calorie goodies but it still represents some serious caloric intake.

So the 3-5 pound window, or whatever you choose, is more for long-term maintenance than the two week full diet break. Basically, if your body weight (and this doesn't include the weight gain from moving back to maintenance) starts to climb by more than 3-5 pounds, you need to clamp down a bit more on your eating habits (or get your exercise plan back on track) before things get out of hand.

In this vein, I want to note that studies of successful dieters note many common behavior patterns but one that is relevant to this chapter is regular monitoring of their body weight. That is, successful dieters tend to keep track of their weight (or body fat) on a regular basis. This could be daily or weekly but keeping regular track tells them when they are slipping and regaining the lost weight/fat so that they can buckle down again. You might contrast this to folks who steadfastly avoid the scale (or always make it a point to wear loose fitting clothes) to avoid the realization that they are getting fat (again). Then they wonder how they 'woke up' fat one day.

If you don't like the scale or body fat measurement, you can simply pick a particular piece of clothing that represents your goal weight/fat level and try it on every so often. If it's getting tight again, you're slipping and it's time to get back on top of your diet and exercising to get back where you need to be.

Again, it's unrealistic for your weight or body fat to be completely unchanging but you're better off getting back on top of your diet and exercise when you've only gained a few pounds than when you've gained a bunch.

Ok, so back to maintenance. As above, a maintenance diet is exactly that, a diet that contains the number of calories (and fulfills other requirements such as protein and essential fatty acids) that will equal your activity level so that your weight/fat level is more or less stable within some range. This is true whether the goal is to perform a full diet break or when a dieter is moving to long term maintenance eating. That's all I'm going to say about this in this chapter, I'll get into more details in the next several chapters. First, more endless words of introduction.

Two different ways to eat at maintenance

As mentioned above, the goal of a full diet break is to eat at maintenance levels. But, to take into account the different types of people reading this book, I'm going to describe two different approaches to moving to maintenance in the next several chapters.

The first approach is aimed at people who really hate counting calories (i.e. most of them). While I'm leery of programs that don't impose some sort of portion control (and note that many popular programs simply hide caloric control while having you count exchanges, or points, or what have you), the simple fact is that most people are not going to keep meticulous track of their food on a day to day basis. So I'm going to give some general eating guidelines that will *tend* to prevent issues with overconsuming calories in either the short or long-term. I'll simply note that if you find your body weight increasing out of the range discussed above, you're going to have to impose some restriction on yourself.

The second approach is for that small minority who is willing to count calories, or at least keep track of their food intake on some level (whether it's portions or what have you). There's more math to determine your daily intake (which is why I suspect most people

63

won't do it) but I think it gives more overall control. I should note that even readers who plan to use the calculation based method in Chapter 15 should still read the next two chapters, as it covers a great deal of information related to food choices and overall meal planning. I'll make a few additional comments on the topic in Chapter 15 as well.

A mixed approach

One approach I've found that is useful is for people who really hate counting calories/portions to spend some time period (say 3-7 days) doing so. That means reading labels, getting out the measuring spoons and cups and generally being miserable and obsessed. The reason for this is that most people are simply atrocious at estimating their food intake.

Studies routinely show that people can underestimate their food intake by 50% (and overestimate their activity by 50% as well). It's not that these folks are lying, most people simply have no conception of what a serving of a given food is. When you get them to actually monitor/measure their food intake, they become far more aware of how much (or little, in some cases) they are actually eating.

Making folks go through the headache of measuring everything for a few days helps them realize not only how much they're eating but what real world portion sizes are. Once they have that established, they can get away with eyeball estimations of their daily intake.

Which is just a longwinded way of saying that some readers may wish to follow the second approach, calculating their requirements and keeping track of everything for some short period of time. This is simply to get an idea of what portions are and about how much food is actually their maintenance level. Once that is established, they can move back to the first approach and sort of eyeball their food intake.

Once again, the ultimate criterion of whether your current food intake (and activity level) constitutes maintenance is what is happening in the real world to your body weight or body fat. Pants getting tighter or the scale going up? No matter what you think you're eating or how much I've suggested as an estimate of your maintenance, you're clearly eating too much for your activity level and need to scale back your food intake, or increase your activity levels, to get your body weight under control.

Moving to maintenance: Fast versus slow

Before I describe the two different approaches to setting up a maintenance diet over the next several chapters, I want to mention that there two different ways to move back to maintenance: fast and slow, which are exactly what they sound like.

In a fast approach, calories are basically ramped up to maintenance quickly over a day or two. This can actually be done in concert with a structured refeed, just make the first day(s) of your refeed the return to maintenance. So start your move to maintenance or the full diet break with a structured refeed, then scale back calories and carbohydrates to maintenance levels for the duration.

The drawbacks to this option is that it's easy to lose control of food intake (what should be a short refeed turns into a long-term binge) and the bloating and water retention can be annoying. Some people also report gastric upset and gas when they ramp up carbs after they haven't been eating any for a while. I think the fast option is probably best for Category 1 dieters (those who aren't under a time crunch) who already have good food control and won't have a problem returning to maintenance after a structured refeed. Category 2 and 3 dieters may still be dealing with changing long-term eating habits and the slow option, described next, is probably better overall.

Which brings us to the other approach to returning to maintenance which is the slow approach. Again, this is exactly what it sounds like, calories are gradually raised to maintenance over some time period (a week at most). Of course, how you go about adding foods back will depend on whether you're using the non-counting/eyeball method described in Chapter 14 or the counting method described in Chapter 15. I'll address this topic individually in each chapter.

I'd say the big advantage of the slow approach is that it avoid major weight spikes which can cause negative psychological effects. The disadvantage is that it's less fun and means you have to be meticulous about your food intake the whole time. Also, from the standpoint of the full diet break, you don't want to take too long to reach maintenance or you won't get the benefits in terms of fixing metabolic rate. At most you should take the first week (of two) to reach maintenance and spend at least 7 days at maintenance levels.

However, this can help with food control, many individuals are completely unaware of what their actual food intake is (or how much, or little, food actually represents maintenance levels) and having to be very aware of their food intake on a day to day basis (at least initially) can act as a teaching tool and help with changing long-term eating habits.

Eating at Maintenance

Non-counting method Part 1

As I mentioned last chapter, I suspect that a majority of readers really don't want to have to count calories on a day to day basis. Certainly not every day for the rest of their life (or even for the 2 weeks of the full diet break). Towards that end, I'm going to offer an approach to eating at maintenance that doesn't require (much) in the way of calculating or calorie tracking.

In this chapter, I'm going to make some general comments about food intake, appetite and caloric intake and in the next chapter I'll give the actual guidelines for setting up a non-counting based maintenance diet.

Yet another warning

I want to make it very clear upfront that I tend to be leery as hell of approaches that rely entirely on the individual to gauge their food intake without monitoring. The reason for this is the number of studies that repeatedly show just how bad people are at it. As mentioned last chapter, people can readily underestimate their food intake by up to 50%, while overestimating their activity by the same 50%.

It's no wonder that people are gaining weight while thinking (and swearing up and down) that they eat very little and burn a ton of calories through exercise. Once again, I'm not saying that folks are lying, people are just really bad at estimating things.

Now, a typical solution to this problem (and the one I'm going to take) is to give a set of eating rules that makes it relatively more difficult to overeat. There are a lot of ways to do it and I'm simply going to present one of them. But note my choice of words two sentences back "relatively more difficult". That's not the same as saying that it's impossible to overeat.

As discussed back in Chapter 3, human body weight tends to be notoriously well regulated and people can easily find themselves gaining back weight even if they appear to be doing everything correctly. Many dieters who have followed the "You don't have to count calories as long as you eat a certain way" types of diets have found out the hard way: either weight loss stalls, or they start regaining weight.

This is one of the big reasons to regularly monitor at least your body weight or body fat (or measure your waist or use some particular piece of clothing to gauge the fit) semi-regularly: it will alert you to when things are sliding. That is, even if you think that you're eating the proper amount, if the scale is creeping back up or that pair of pants is fitting tighter, clearly you are in a calorie surplus. That's true even if you follow the guidelines I'm going to give.

This is yet another reason that you may wish to spend at least some time measuring and weighing foods when you eat them, to get a better idea of what portions actually are relative to what you think they are. I'll mention this below and, unfortunately, make one very serious recommendation about something you really should measure.

The effects of nutrients on spontaneous food intake

Ok, first I should probably define what is meant in the section heading by 'spontaneous food intake'. Basically, that phrase refers to the amount of food that people will eat if left to their own devices, that is they aren't monitoring their total food intake at all.

This is an important concept as different foods tend to affect spontaneous food intake a bit differently. With the exception of some of the goofier diet schemes out there, most of the "Eat all you want but don't worry about counting calories" approaches recommend that dieters eat in such a way that spontaneous food intake is automatically reduced.

Quite in fact, this is the basic theory behind both low-fat AND low-carbohydrate diets (I'm ignoring the idea of a metabolic advantage inherent to low-carb diets, that's a can of worms I don't want to address here). Which probably confused the heck out of everyone, so let me explain.

A great many studies have shown that high fat diets (lets ignore the meaninglessness of that term) tend to promote what researchers call passive overconsumption of calories. Translated into non-gibberish, that means that when you give people access to high fat foods, they tend to eat more at a given meal without noticing it. Hence passive overconsumption. The essential problem is that, in the short-term (over a meal), fat doesn't blunt hunger or alter food intake.

So the logic goes, if people reduce fat intake, they'll end up eating fewer calories and lose weight. That's it, the whole premise was more or less based around the idea that if people eat less fat, they'll eat fewer calories and lose weight. This wasn't the only reason, mind you, but it was one of the main ones.

And this is true to a small degree although the effect amounts to very little in the long run. It's been estimated that for every 1% reduction in fat intake, you will lose a whopping 1.6 grams of weight per day. Which, over the range that people can realistically reduce fat intake adds up to almost nothing, maybe 5-10 pounds lost over 6 months which is nothing to write home about. This also assumes that people don't just eat more of the other foods. Which turns out to be a rather incorrect assumption in the real world.

Additionally, there's a limit to how far fat can be reduced before the diet tastes like cardboard and people won't follow it (some research has found better dietary compliance to moderate compared to very low fat-diets). As well, people on low-fat diets, just like everyone else, often start to regain weight even if they keep fat intake low. Why? Because they start to eat more of the foods that they are allowed.

None of this was helped by the fact that when the low-fat craze came about, food companies rushed high calorie but low or nonfat foods (Snackwell's anybody?) to market. Since people figured that all they had to pay attention to was fat intake, they ended up overeating anyway (by eating high calorie but low- or nonfat foods).

So how can the same basic idea apply to low-carbohydrate diets? First let me say that numerous studies have shown that spontaneous food intake on low-carbohydrate (also called ketogenic diets) goes down. There's a few reasons for this. Perhaps the primary one is that when you remove an entire category of food (carbohydrates) that happens to make up 50% or more of people's food intakes, they pretty much can't help but eat less. As well, since protein turns out to have the largest effect on hunger blunting, the high protein intake tended to help as well (as least one researcher thinks that the benefits of low-carb diets are occurring because people typically increase their protein intake on such diets). The fat intake also tends to keep people full in the long-run which seems to contradict what I wrote above about spontaneous food intake but I'll explain in a second.

Additionally, for people who don't handle carbohydrates well (because they are insulin resistant), high carbohydrate intakes tend to spike and crash blood glucose, making them feel lethargic and hungry. Low-carbohydrate/high-protein diets tend to stabilize blood glucose in these folks and the blood sugar crash induced hunger goes away. Finally, ketones (which are produced by the liver when carbohydrates are taken below a certain level) may blunt hunger, although the evidence for that effect isn't great.

Of course, while this works in the short-term, anybody who's been on a low-carbohydrate diet for any period of time realizes that the same type of effect as with low-fat eventually occurs. Either weight loss stalls or starts climbing again. The reasons are similar to what happens on low-fat diets: people start eating more of the foods that they are allowed. As well, the high fat intake of most low-carbohydrate diets can come back to bite people in the ass, they end up gorging on high-fat foods and eating a lot of calories. As well, companies are now rushing low-carb (but high-calorie) foods to market which is going to lead people down the same road as what happened with low-fat. Focused only on carbohydrate content, they'll end up overeating and either not lose weight or end up gaining it.

And that's how both low-fat and low-carb diets are predicated on the basic idea that, by altering your food intake, people will spontaneously eat less and lose weight. I should note that at least one recent study has shown that diets higher in protein (25% vs.12% of total calories) found a similar effect: the subjects in the higher protein group automatically ate less and lost weight/fat.

I suppose I should mention alcohol since it is a nutrient (of sorts) that people consume. Unfortunately, the effects of alcohol on spontaneous food intake and body weight are a little bit schizophrenic. In men increasing alcohol intake tends to cause an increase in body weight (measured by BMI); in women, increasing alcohol tends to be associated with a decreased body weight. The reasons are still up to debate but, as much as anything, it's probably that men tend to eat (and eat fatty foods) when they drink while women tend to drink instead of eating.

How nutrients affect satiety and satiation

Ok, I know I threw a couple more big words at you up there so let me explain them briefly. Satiety is basically short-term hunger, over the course of a meal or so; satiation has to do with longer-term hunger (more accurately called appetite). This is an important distinction to make because each nutrient affects things a bit differently.

As I mentioned above, dietary fat tends to have almost no effect in the short-term, which is why we get the effect of passive overconsumption. In contrast, both protein and carbohydrate tend to blunt hunger in the short-term. Now I want to comment that I think the studies in question are a little bit goofy. Typically, they use what is called a pre-load design, subjects are given a snack (containing various amounts of the nutrients) and then allowed an all you can eat buffet about 30 minutes later. Researchers look at the food intake at the buffet and draw some (in my mind, poor) conclusions about real world food intake.

Ignoring every other issue with these studies, one of the most important is that they only look at a single meal. I bring this up because how much you eat over a span of 24 hours (or days) is arguably more important. And how much you eat over a day depends to some degree on how long you go between meals. Ultimately, a study looking at a single meal (especially using a preload design) tells us little about real world eating behavior.

I bring this up because, as anybody who has followed an extremely low-fat diet knows, dietary fat tends to keep you from getting hungry as soon. Readers may be familiar with the idea of a meal that 'sticks to their ribs', an old folk saying referring to how long certain foods sit in the stomach. Higher fat intakes (up to a point) make food sit in the gut longer, and that tends to keep people fuller in the long-term.

Within the context of the typical low-fat diet, this is made even more pronounced when the diet is low in fiber (which slows the rate at which food leaves the stomach) and high in refined carbohydrates (the ones that people like to eat). Add to that frequently insufficient protein, you get a lot of carbs hitting the bloodstream very rapidly, first spiking and then crashing blood glucose which tends to promote hunger. In many dieters (note again to my critics: I didn't say all people), extremely low-fat intakes, especially when they are coupled with low-fiber, low-protein and refined carbohydrates make people hungrier. I want to point out that this has as much to do with an incorrect diet setup as with the concept of the high-carbohydrate diet itself. People who get sufficient protein, and some dietary fat, along with choosing the less refined carbohydrates often do just fine with such a diet. But I digress.

You can easily test the effect of dietary fat on appetite yourself. First eat something like a bagel or some other fairly refined carbohydrate plain. See how soon you are hungry again. If you're like most people, it will be fairly soon, an hour or two at the most. Now eat that same bagel with 1/2-1 tablespoon of peanut butter on it and see how much longer you stay full. Between the protein content of the peanut butter and the fat content, the entire combination will stay in your stomach longer, promoting fullness. As well, the fat and protein will tend to slow the entry of glucose into the bloodstream, avoiding major blood glucose swings and crashes.

Basically, dietary fat is sort of a double-edged sword when it comes to caloric intake, satiety and satiation. High dietary fat intakes tend to promote excessive caloric intakes via the passive overconsumption effects; very low fat intakes tend to leave people hungrier sooner (especially when combined with a diet of highly refined carbohydrates and too little protein and fiber) and they end up eating more as well.

This argues for a moderate fat intake (20-25% of total calories, I'll explain more next chapter) as probably being optimal and some recent research supports that idea; moderate fat diets tend to have better dietary adherence and improve health more so than extremely low or high fat diets. Moderate dietary fat intakes also appear to give an optimal effect in terms of slowing glucose release into the bloodstream and moderating blood glucose levels.

I already mentioned above that protein has been found to have the greatest impact on hunger. In the short-term studies, carbs come in second and fat is last. Over the longer term, whether carbs or fat is superior sort of depends. Unrefined naturally occurring carbohydrates tend to keep people fairly full, especially when combined with protein, fat and fiber but the more highly refined carbohydrates (i.e. the ones people are actually eating in the real world) seem to stimulate hunger more often than not. Between a fast rate of digestion and everything that accompanies it, highly refined carbs can cause more problems than they solve.

Ending the Diet Approach 1
Non-counting method Part 2

In the last chapter, I introduced some general concepts about how protein, carbs and fat can spontaneously affect caloric intake. That directly leads into this chapter which will list some general guidelines and explain how to put it all together to develop a maintenance level diet that doesn't require you to count and measure every morsel of food.

Eating guidelines

After the last chapter, you should already have a pretty decent idea of what I'm going to suggest in this chapter. Below, I'm going to list a series of 'rules' for eating that will tend to make strict calorie counting 'mostly' unnecessary. It encompasses what I discussed last chapter and adds a few more helpful hints. I'll address each in more detail in a second and then explain how to put this into practice.

Basic Eating Rules

1. Eat more frequently
2. Eat plenty of lean protein
3. Eat a moderate amount of fat at each meal
4. Eat plenty of fiber from vegetables, fruits, and unrefined carbohydrates like beans
5. Eat moderate amounts of refined carbohydrates such as breads, pasta, rice and grains
6. Eat slowly
7. Continue to utilize free meals and/or structured refeeds
8. Exercise

73

Eat more frequently

A good bit of research had found that eating more frequently (while splitting your total daily caloric intake) keeps hunger better under control and this is true in both lean and obese individuals (for whom hunger/appetite control can be a real problem). There are a number of reasons for this. Perhaps the biggest one is avoiding extreme hunger which can occur when meals are spaced out too far. This occurs for a number of reasons but decreasing blood glucose is one of them. I'm sure every reader can identify with waiting too long to eat, feeling lightheaded and ending up at the candy machine ravenous.

As an additional benefit, eating smaller meals overall has an effect on the stomach's stretchability, decreasing it over time. Basically, when you eat lots of large meals all of the time, the stomach stretches more. In that the physical stretching of the stomach is one of many signals for fullness, a stomach that is less easily stretched tends to fill up faster and let you know that you're full.

Now, I should mention that some earlier research suggested that snacking had the opposite effect, increasing caloric intake and causing weight gain. But this research was really looking at what happens when you add snacks (and I suspect the typical types of junk food snacks) to a normal diet; it wasn't looking at what happens when you split your normal daily food intake into more, smaller meals.

It's the latter goal that I'm describing: splitting your daily food intake into smaller meals. Now, bodybuilders and athletes are used to eating 5-6 (or more) meals per day and take it as part of the price they pay. But this may not be possible for all readers. Job, life, etc. all get in the way. While it might be ideal to eat 5-6 mini-meals per day, this isn't always realistic.

Now, I can't know what type of diet my readers are on or how frequently they are eating. So I'll simply say that a total daily meal frequency of 4-6 'meals' per day is probably reasonable while on a maintenance intake diet. We might reasonably figure 5 as a realistic number which would mean breakfast, lunch, and dinner with a couple of small snacks in-between them. I want to make it very clear that all snacks and in-between meals should more or less follow the other rules I'm going to describe as much as possible (getting fiber with a lot of snacks can be a problem but do your best).

That means that an ideal snack should contain protein, a moderate amount of fat, some fiber and the rest. Translation: a plain bagel is not a meal, a piece of fruit is not a meal, a candy bar surely isn't a meal. A bagel with a bit of mustard, mayo or cheese and some turkey qualifies, a piece of fruit with a glass of low fat milk qualifies, even some of the meal replacement bars (try to pick the ones that have reasonable amounts of protein, carbs and fat) is workable. Would it be ideal to eat a small whole food meal containing protein, fat, fiber and the rest at each meal? Yes. Is that realistic for everyone? No.

Eat plenty of lean protein

As I mentioned last chapter, protein has the greatest effect on blunting hunger, beating out both fat and carbohydrates. As well, recent research is also showing that a higher protein intake after a diet tends to limit weight gain and the weight that is gained tends to be lean body mass. Frankly, if there's a single problem I have with many diets, it's that they are too low in protein. This tends to be especially true of high-carbohydrate diets with moderate carb diets (such as The Zone) and low-carbohydrate diets typically providing more than enough protein.

Every meal eaten while at maintenance must contain a source of protein and this will go a long way towards keeping caloric intake at bay. I guess the question is how much. Somewhere between 3-6 ounces (21-42 grams of protein or so) depending on body weight is probably a good rule of thumb with lighter individuals eating the smaller amounts and heavier individuals more. To put this in perspective, 3 ounces of protein is about the amount that would fit in your cupped palm, it is also about the same size as a deck of cards. Most restaurants will typically serve you at least twice that much. A list of good lean protein sources appears in below.

Lean protein sources

Skinless chicken breast

Low-fat fish: tuna, cod, halibut, flounder, lobster, crab

Extremely lean red meat

Low or nonfat dairy

Egg whites with limited whole eggs

Beef jerky

Some of the fattier cuts of red meat can also be eaten in moderation, the same goes for whole eggs (see comments about fat intake below). As I mentioned previously, research is finding that higher calcium intakes, especially from dairy sources, has benefits in terms of body fat and body weight levels. Consuming low or nonfat dairy products as part of a maintenance diet is a good idea. I mention protein powder as they are a staple of athletes and bodybuilders and are coming more into vogue outside of those populations. While I would prefer to see people eat whole foods, using powders in a limited fashion can be another way to ensure adequate protein intake while eating at maintenance.

Eat a moderate amount of fat at each meal

There is a growing amount of research suggesting that moderate fat diets (about 25% of total calories) are more effective, as well as being healthier, than either extremely low or extremely high-fat diets. There are a number of reasons for this, none of which I'm going to bother getting into.

I haven't talked much about dietary fat except for a few brief comments back in Chapter 6. Without going into huge amounts of detail, let me say that there are 4 different types of dietary fat you need to be familiar with. The first are the trans-fatty acids which have received a good deal of negative press lately, and for good reason. These are a man-made fat, found in almost all processed foods (they are often listed as partially hydrogenated vegetable oils) that really have no place in any healthy diet.

The second type are saturated fats; found primarily in animal products, saturated fats are solid at room temperature. In general, saturated fat intake should be limited for health reasons. However, it's nearly impossible to avoid them completely.

The third type are monounsaturated fats, of which olive oil is probably the best known. From a health perspective, olive oil is at least neutral and may very well be beneficial. Monounsaturates should make up the majority of your fat intake.

Finally are the polyunsaturates which are also known as essential fatty acids (because they are essential to get from the diet); they are liquid at room temperature. I don't want to get into complicated details but there are two primary 'classes' of polyunsaturates referred to as omega-6 (w-6) and omega-3 (w-3) fatty acids. W-6 fatty acids are found pretty readily in our food supply while w-3 are not. Recent research has found that w-3 fatty acids (of which the fish oils are probably the most talked about) have profound health benefits and I think it's important to ensure w-3 intake on any diet. My preferred option is to take 6X1 grams fish oil capsules per day; an alternative option (for people who hate taking pills or don't like fishy burps that the pills can cause) is to consume 1 tablespoon of flax oil per day.

Once again, it would be ideal if the majority of your dietary fat came from monounsaturated fat (think oil and vinegar dressing on your salads) while ensuring your essential fatty acid intake; the remainder of your fat would come from saturated fats which are basically impossible to avoid.

Ok, so what about amounts, what constitutes a moderate fat intake as far as a maintenance diet is concerned? I think 10-14 grams per meal or thereabouts is about right although smaller snacks may need less (say 5-7 grams of fat). Ok, now I know that I originally said that you wouldn't have to count or measure stuff but this is a place where I'm going to go back on that.

So you won't skip it, right now I want you go to your kitchen and get out a bottle of vegetable oil (or oil and vinegar salad dressing or something) and a tablespoon measure. Ok, pour the oil into the tablespoon. That's 14 grams of fat right there, that's the maximum you can have at each meal. Right, not very much. Now you see another reason that it's easy to overconsume dietary fat, very very little fat contains a ton of calories. I strongly (STRONGLY) advise you to measure your fat intake while eating at maintenance, at least for a bit. Eyeballing it or estimating it is almost sure to get you into trouble calorie wise.

Now, depending on your other foods choices (especially protein), your meals will probably contain some amount of dietary fat to begin with. This can range from almost none to quite a bit depending on what you eat. Again, this means that you really need to keep track of how much fat you're getting. As a general rule, I'd say this: if your other food choices (such as low-fat dairy or other proteins) contain dietary fat, don't add any more to the meal. Odds are there is already enough. If your other foods contain little to no fat (think lean chicken breast or nonfat dairy), you should add a small amount of dietary fat to the meal. Throw some oil and vinegar dressing on your salad or something like that.

Eat plenty of fiber from fruits, vegetables and unrefined carbohydrates such as beans

The benefits of fiber go far beyond health, it is a potent aid to both weight loss and maintenance eating. The reason is that fiber (well, certain types of fiber) keep food in the stomach longer, promoting fullness. Additionally, that same fiber takes up quite a bit of room in the stomach and the physical stretching of the stomach is one (of many) signals for fullness. As well, fiber is chewy and takes time to eat, meals high in fiber tend to automatically slow down your eating, giving your brain time to register that you're full.

Finally, the foods high in fiber (fruits, vegetables, naturally occurring carbs like beans and such) are also high in nutrients, both vitamins and minerals that are required for health, as well as a class of nutrients called phytonutrients which are turning out to have numerous health benefits. Once again, your grandmother was right, eat your fruits and vegetables. I should add that some mainstream nutrition types would include the higher fiber grains in this category and this may be true if you're talking about some of the coarser breads. But the more you refine a food, the more fiber you remove and the less nutritious it tends to become. So I'm putting all refined grains in the category of food described in the next section.

Now, while most vegetables (with the exception of the starchy vegetables mentioned previously) have so few calories that they can basically be eaten without limit, this isn't the case for the other foods in this category. The usual issue, as with beans below, has more to do with the toppings people put on top of their veggies; melted cheese is common and many salad dressings contain a considerable amount of calories as either carbohydrates, fats, or both.

While difficult, it is conceivable to overeat fruits, especially if you go with stuff like grapes and raisins. Dried fruit is a nightmare (by removing the water content, you remove most of the bulk and fiber) calorically, canned fruit almost always has extra sugar added and I think fruit juice is horrid food from most standpoints. You've taken out the bulk and the fiber and managed to concentrate the calories horribly. So go to your produce section in the grocery store and stick with whole fruits and that means eating the skins (where the fiber is) too. As I'll mention below, a single piece of fruit makes a good addition to your normal meals and, unless you go really nuts, you'll be hard pressed to overeat fruit.

The naturally occurring carbohydrate foods such as beans (or legumes, if you prefer) and potatoes can be a bit more problematic. While it's unlikely that most people would drastically overconsume such foods, it is a possibility so be aware. But both are high in fiber (make sure and eat the skin on the potato) and bulk so they will tend to limit their own intake. Perhaps a bigger issue is what people tend to put on such foods as toppings.

A baked potato by itself (or with something like ketchup, my preference, or fat free ranch dressing or salsa) is one thing, a potato smothered in butter and sour cream (how most people eat it) is another entirely. Bean salads are often swimming in oil and people often bury all of the above foods (ok, not fruit) in high fat cheese more often than not.

Finally are nuts which I suppose belong in this category. Although unrefined and a good source of protein and healthy fats, nuts can be extremely easy to over-consume and it doesn't take many to contribute a really monstrous number of calories. If you choose to eat them, they should be measured (similarly to your fat intake).

Eat moderate amounts of refined carbohydrates such as breads, pasta, rice and grains

Now the carb freaks and mainstream nutritionists will take issue with what I'm going to write here but that's tough, it's my book. While the dogma about such foods is that they are wonderful for health, impossible to overeat and all that crap (and this may be true in the artificial world of the lab and under some very specific circumstances), in the real world this just doesn't turn out to be the case.

A great many people (note to critics with poor reading comprehension: I didn't say ALL people) can readily overconsume such foods. And the fact is that they can be somewhat energy dense (meaning they contain a lot of calories in small bulk). If you don't believe me, go get a box of pasta and look at just how little pasta makes a one or three ounce serving.

Now cook it up and compare that to what you probably would typically eat if you had pasta for dinner; you'd probably eat twice or three times the standard 'serving' size to the tune of many hundreds of calories. And that's before you add the toppings, which may range from inconsequential like marinara sauce, to the high fat cream sauces and cheese. The same comment goes for rice or any food in that category. Or check most of the commercial cereals sometime, the standard serving and what most people actually eat have nothing in common.

In the US especially, the serving sizes of grain based foods such as bagels and muffins has exploded. While a bagel or muffin may have only contained a couple of hundred calories in previous years, calorie counts of 400 or more calories is not uncommon for the supersized versions. Bread in and of itself usually isn't a huge issue, a slice is usually only so large (unless you're eating Texas toast which is huge) and most people won't eat that many slices in a single sitting.

Perhaps a larger problem comes when you add these types of foods to the rest of the modern diet: super high in fat, and low in fiber. Add to that insulin resistance that is common with inactive individuals who are overweight and you get into problems. Even marginally refined grains can do bad things to blood glucose and studies are clearly showing that reducing total carbohydrate intake and increasing protein intake is better for insulin resistant individuals from a variety of standpoints including blood glucose levels and health.

Now, the point of my comments is not to say that these types of foods are totally off limits (which is an extreme that some nutrition experts reach), simply that they can be more problematic than fruits, vegetables and the naturally occurring carbohydrates for a variety of reasons. This is yet another place that I'd highly suggest (though not as strongly as for dietary fat) that you spend a bit of time getting familiar with serving sizes on any of the foods that you wish to eat. Which is to say that serving of pasta or rice or what have you is ok, just don't go crazy with it. Eating a monster bowl of pasta or rice is going to add hundreds and hundreds of calories to your daily intake without you even noticing it. A good rule of thumb might be to limit your starchy carbohydrates at any given meal to the amount that would fit in a cupped palm (just like protein above) or slightly more.

I should mention that some individuals run into problems with even the smallest amount of grains in their diet. These are usually fatter individuals (high end of diet Category 2 or those still in Category 3) who are severely insulin resistant. In that case, grains may simply have to be eliminated completely. Which means that fruits, vegetables, and the few naturally occurring starches like potatoes and yams will be the only carbohydrates allowed.

Eat slowly

Yet another place where everyone's grandmother was correct about eating. From a satiety/fullness standpoint, eating more slowly is beneficial. The reason is that there is a delay between eating and when your brain gets the 'signal' (which is sent via nerves and chemicals in your bloodstream) that you are full. On average, the delay is about 20 minutes or so although even this may be impaired in some individuals. The point being that if you eat super quickly, you will tend to eat more than if you take your time. This is one advantage of high-fiber foods, especially salad; they take time to eat. Not surprisingly, a recent study found that people who ate a salad first ate less during the normal meal. Who'd have guessed? I mean other than just about everybody.

Continue to utilize free meals and/or refeeds

Although the goal of maintenance is, well, maintenance, I still think continuing with free meals as part of your overall structure is a very good idea. That is, even though the recommendations in this chapter are somewhat free form, there are still restrictions in terms of what you can and can't eat (i.e. you can't eat anything you want in unlimited amounts). Allowing for a free meal or two each week will go a long way psychologically to sticking with the other dietary habits you're trying to maintain. The guidelines provided previously still apply.

For someone looking at long-term maintenance, I also think that refeeds can be utilized, as described in previous chapters. For the full diet break, a refeed really isn't appropriate except possibly to start the move to maintenance as described two chapters back.

Exercise

Except for helping you decide a few of the parameters of what I talked about in this booklet, I didn't really talk that much about exercise and this isn't the place to get into huge amounts of detail on the topic. I'll only say (and this is discussed in greater detail in The Rapid Fat Loss Handbook) that most research suggests that realistic amounts of exercise has a limited ability to really impact on total weight loss. Some of it suggests that exercise can shift the proportions of what is lost, however; exercisers tend to lose more fat and less lean body mass. Additionally, some studies suggest that adding exercise to a diet can improve dietary adherence; exercisers stick to their diet more effectively.

Perhaps more importantly, at least within the context of eating at maintenance, a good deal of research suggests that the primary role of exercise is in maintaining weight loss/preventing weight regain. There are a few reasons for this. One is that exercise helps to cancel out some of the diet induced reduction in metabolic rate that can promote weight regain. As well, there tends to be a decrease in resting fat oxidation after the diet, exercise can also correct this defect. As mentioned, some research suggests that exercise can increase dietary compliance.

Psychologically, many people seem to link their eating and exercise habits: they tend to be more aware of their eating and strive to eat healthier when they are exercising. I should note that some people take an opposite approach: figuring that they are burning far more calories than they are, they assume that they have earned the double cheeseburger and milkshake after a workout and end up eating too much.

In any event, if you aren't already on an exercise program, while you're eating at maintenance is an excellent time to start. I can't get into all of the details necessary to set up an exercise program in this booklet. You can either check out one of the million and one books on the topic or get my first book The Ketogenic Diet which addresses the issue in some detail. I will say that I think a proper exercise program should contain some mix of resistance exercise (weight training) and cardiovascular or aerobic training.

I should note that the research on this topic tends to find that quite a bit of exercise, about 2500 calories/week is necessary to completely prevent weight regain. Lesser amounts will prevent some of the weight regain but not all of it. Now, this is quite a bit of activity and that is a consideration. To put it into perspective, the average person can burn about 10 calories per minute during a moderate intensity aerobic activity, less if they work at a lower intensity. To burn 2500 calories per week amounts to 400 calories per day if they exercise 6 days per week and progressively more if they exercise fewer days.

This means that about a minimum of of 45 minutes (if you're willing to work fairly hard) or up to 90 minutes per day of exercise may be needed to accumulate that 2500 calories/week. Simply keep that in mind when you set up an exercise program. Walking for 20 minutes a few times per week simply isn't going to cut it.

Putting it all together

Ok, now I have a problem which I've alluded to previously: I have no idea what kind of diet you may be following as you decide to do a full diet break. As I mentioned, when I first wrote these chapters, they were mainly within the context of the crash diet described in my other booklet; I'm having to change a lot of stuff on the fly to adapt it. This explains why there are some rather abrupt and brief bits of info above; it's information that was covered in-depth in the other booklet but not in this one.

The basic diet/meal plan I've described above has every meal containing an ample amount of lean protein, a controlled/moderate amount of fat, an unlimited amount of vegetables, some fruits and a controlled amount of concentrated carbohydrates (starches). Frankly, ignoring all of the myriad issues that I'd normally consider when deciding what I think is the 'optimal' diet for a given individual, I think that type of diet is about as close to ideal as we are going to get.

The issue is how to reach that ideal and what changes need to be made and that depends entirely on what type of diet you're moving from. Someone coming off of a low-carbohydrate diet, who is eating primarily protein and fat (and hopefully some vegetables) is probably going to apply the information I presented above a little bit differently than someone on a Zone type of high-carbohydrate/low fat diet. So let's look at each one briefly (don't forget that you can move to maintenance in either a slow or fast fashion as described last chapter).

First up, low-carbohydrate diets. Depending on the flavor, the typical low-carbohydrate diet such as Atkins, Protein Power or South Beach has dieters eating quite a bit of protein, a lot of vegetables and quite varying amounts of fat (the more recent trend with low-carbohydrate diets is to avoid the uncontrolled fat intake of the original Atkins diet, and also focus on fat quality; something I see as a move in the right direction). Moving to the diet described isn't very difficult. Protein intake will generally remain unchanged, although leaner protein sources may need to be chosen to moderate fat intake. Hopefully, low-carbohydrate dieters are already eating lots of high-fiber veggies. They may have to modify what they top those vegetables with: full fat cheeses and the low-carbohydrate salad dressings (which are typically very high in fat) won't cut it. Low-fat cheeses or light versions of salad dressings work just fine. So does oil and vinegar.

Remember from last chapter that one of the requirements for the diet break is that you eat at least 100 grams of carbohydrate per day. If you're in a situation where you know that even small amounts of grains or starches cause you problems, then fruit is probably the best choice. Four average sized apples or bananas will contain 100 grams of carbohydrates easily. Just add a piece of fruit to each meal.

Depending on which 'flavor' of low-carbohydrate diet someone is on, they may have to make some rather severe adjustments to both the quantity and quality of their fat intake. Some of the popular low-carb diets pretty much tell people to eat what they want with no attention to details of fat quantity or quality. During the move to maintenance, maintaining those types of eating behaviors is a recipe for disaster and I highly recommend that folks start paying attention to the amounts and types of fat that they are consuming. Yes, this means reading labels. Yes, this is a huge pain in the ass. But in the long run it will do a tremendous amount of good in terms of the success of your full diet break (or move to maintenance). Obviously, folks on those flavors of low-carbohydrate diets that limit dietary fat intake (or at least pay lip-service to the concept of fat quality) don't need to be as concerned although they may still want to track quantities to some degree when they do a diet break/move to maintenance.

Next up are the moderate carbohydrate/moderate fat diets such as the Zone or 40/30/30 nutrition or Dan Duchaine's Isocaloric diet. While specifics vary, most of these diets are set up around sufficient protein intakes with moderate amounts of carbs and fat. All invariably end up being calorically restricted because of the way that they are set up but most also put an emphasis on eating a lot of unrefined carbohydrates, especially fruits and vegetables (and low glycemic index starches) as well as healthier fats. Frankly, again ignoring a lot of variability, if I had to choose a single dietary approach as being close to ideal for most people, these types of diets are probably close to it.

If I worked out the contributions of the different nutrients for my proposed non-counting maintenance diet, they would end up very close to the already existing moderate carb/fat diets. The main modification that folks on these types of diets need to make is simply to increase total caloric intake, via carbohydrates and fats (protein intake is usually sufficient to begin with). Yes, I know, that takes you out of the magic percentage ratios but I don't think it matters. Simply add foods as necessary (even some of the, gasp, concentrated starches). Getting 100 grams of carbohydrates shouldn't be a problem.

Finally are high-carbohydrate, low-fat diets. Frankly, these vary so much that it's very difficult for me to set out a standard. I will only say that, in my experience, many non-bodybuilder/athlete high-carbohydrate diets tend to be lower in protein than I think is ideal from either a dieting or maintenance standpoint. So some high-carb dieters will need to make a real effort to increase lean protein intake to meet my recommendations above.

As well, low-fat is one of those terms that can vary quite significantly. Technically, any diet that contains less than 30% of total calories is a low-fat diet but I find many low-fat dieters cutting dietary fat as low as they can get it; I've seen 10% or lower in some cases. As I mentioned above, research is finding that moderate fat diets (in the range of 25% of total calories) are probably healthier, taste better, and have better adherence. So extreme low-fat dieters may need to raise fat intake to moderate levels, emphasizing healthy fats such as the monounsaturates (and ensuring that they get their fish oils or flax). Carbohydrate intake is usually more than sufficient that I don't see any real need to alter it. Just make sure that you're getting plenty of high-fiber veggies, some fruits, and trying to avoid the super refined grains if you're on such a diet.

And then there's everything else, the thousands of diets that don't fit into any neat category. Obviously I can't address all of them, I doubt I'm familiar with all of them in the first place. All I can say is that you should compare your current dietary intake to what I describe above as my ideal non-counting maintenance diet and adjust as necessary. If you're having major problems, drop me an email telling me what the diet is on you're on and I can probably give you some guidance in terms of what to adjust.

84

Eating at Maintenance

Calculation method

So now you've read through some suggestions in the last two chapters on how to move to maintenance without the need to strictly count or control portions. But perhaps you're one of those individuals who wants or simply needs more control than that. Or maybe you tried maintaining your weight without tracking portions, it didn't work and you want to calculate, weigh and measure everything for some period of time. This chapter will tell you how to do that.

I want to warn you up front (this is for any particularly critical readers) that I'm having to simplify a lot of information in this chapter. Frankly, this chapter and the last three have been a huge headache for me, trying to write something that isn't super complicated but which I am satisfied with in terms of the recommendations I want to give.

The fundamental problem is that I don't think any single diet is appropriate for everyone, what may be ideal depends on such issues as body fat, gender, genetics, food preferences, insulin sensitivity, exercise patterns and a whole host of other topics. When I consult on people's diets, I may have to ask them a dozen or more questions to get a rough idea of what I think might be ideal for them. Even that usually has to be tweaked.

My point being that this chapter is sort of a simplified version of the thought processes I would typically go through in setting up a diet for someone (or myself). It would take the better part of another book (yes, a future book project) to put all of the variables down so I'm sort of copping out here and giving the abbreviated version of how I would approach this topic.

Finally, I want to point out that while you're going to have to do some calculations involving calorie values, you won't be counting calories per se during maintenance. Rather, you'll be counting grams of each nutrient. Which, while the same as counting calories seems not to give people the same headache or anxiety as strict calorie counting. I mean, anybody should be able to look at food label package and pull off the protein, carbs, fat and fiber grams to fill them into daily or meal totals. I hope so anyhow.

I should mention again that, as with the previous chapters, this was originally written for people moving off of the diet described in my <u>Rapid Fat Loss Handbook</u>. Which is to say that it won't (and really can't) take into account the specific diet that you're on. Rather, it's going to give a set of generalized recommendations based on what I think a good maintenance diet should look like (essentially it's a calculated version of what I described last chapter).

Step 1: Determine maintenance calorie levels

The first and most important step in developing a maintenance level diet is to determine maintenance calorie levels. By definition, your maintenance calorie level represents the number of calories per day that you need to maintain your current weight or body fat. Again note that exacting body weight/fat maintenance with zero fluctuation is an unrealistic pipe dream. We're going to be a bit more flexible and let maintenance calorie levels be a level that keeps your weight/fat within some range.

What this means is that we need to get an estimate of what your total daily calorie expenditure might be. This represents the sum total of calories burned due to basal metabolic rate (BMR), the thermic effect of activity (TEA) and the thermic effect of food (TEF). Lately, researchers have been dividing up the activity component into an exercise component and something they call NEAT (non-exercise activity thermogenesis) which includes all daily movement or activity that isn't formal exercise. Schematically, your total daily energy expenditure could be written as

$$\text{Total energy expenditure (TEE)} = \text{BMR} + \text{TEF} + \text{TEA} + \text{NEAT}$$

As the name suggests BMR represents the number of calories your body burns at rest. TEA represents calories burned during exercise. TEF represents the number of calories that are burned in processing food (digestion, storage, etc.). Finally is NEAT which, as I mentioned, compromises all daily activities that aren't exercise.

I should mention that the most variable parts of the above equation are TEA and NEAT which can both vary quite significantly between individuals. BMR and TEF tend to be fairly consistent. For example, a sedentary individual may burn effectively zero calories per day in formal exercise while an elite athlete may burn several thousand. It's turning out that NEAT is very individual and can vary quite a bit; some people burn a lot of calories spontaneously throughout the day just moving around while others don't. This appears to explain some of the rather large differences in weight gain when you overfeed people, some of them ramp up NEAT, burning off a lot of the calories while others do no such thing. The second group gets fat rather readily while the first does not.

We are going to use some rather standard estimates for each of those three components, adjust it for metabolic rate slowdown due to dieting and use that as an estimate of your maintenance caloric requirement. Unfortunately, there's no easy way to measure NEAT at this point so you'll just have to sort of build it into the estimate you make in a second.

Please note my use of the word estimate as that is all these values are; do not take them as holy writ. Based on a number of different variables, total daily energy expenditure can have some variance and you may have to make adjustments to your daily caloric intake depending on real world changes in body weight and body fat (which means you need to monitor them to some degree).

Quite simply, if you're regaining weight (this doesn't include the rapid water weight gain that accompanies high carb or salt intakes), you need to cut your calories back a bit; if you're still losing at supposed 'maintenance' levels, you need to increase calories slightly.

Depending on activity levels, total daily energy expenditure usually ranges from about 12 calories per pound of body weight for relatively sedentary individuals to 15-16 calories per pound for relatively average activity levels (3-4 hours/week of exercise plus normal daily activity) with extremely active individuals (think endurance athletes training 2 or more hours per day) going up to 20 cal/lb or more.

This means that, on average, a multiplier of 12-16 calories per pound of total body weight is about right (with highly trained athletes going higher) to estimate maintenance. Because dieting slows the metabolism somewhat, we're going to adjust that down by about 10% to account for metabolic slowdown giving a range of 11-15 calories per pound or so. Use table 1 on the next page to select your body weight multiplier. The category descriptions appear below.

Sedentary means no activity other than sitting at a desk (or light household activity). Lightly active would include low intensity aerobic activity. Moderate activity would be either higher intensity aerobic activity or weight training, very active would be a combination of weight training (3+ times/week) and aerobics and extremely active is reserved for athletes in training, individuals training 2 or more hours per day. So use those descriptions as guidelines for picking your body weight multiplier. In general, women (who typically have a lower metabolic rate to start with) should use the lower value, men the higher value.

Table 1: Body weight multiplier to estimate current maintenance

Description	Body weight multiplier (cal/lb)
Sedentary	10-11
Lightly active	11-12
Moderately active	12-13
Very active	14-15
Extremely active	18-19

Ok, first annoying math step, I need you to multiply your current weight in pounds by the above multiplication factor to get your total daily calories per day. Once again, metric readers should multiply their weight in kilograms by 2.2 to get pounds.

$$\underline{\hspace{2cm}} * \underline{\hspace{2cm}} = \underline{\hspace{2cm}}$$
Weight   Multiplier   Calories/day

This is your estimated caloric requirement per day to maintain you body weight.

A quick tangent: the Atwater factors

So what in the holy hell, you ask, are the Atwater factors. They are the values I suspect most dieters are already familiar, representing the caloric value of the different nutrients. You'll be using them below to calculate caloric intakes from the various nutrients which is why I'm presenting them here. They appear in table 2 below.

Table 2: Atwater factors

Nutrient	Calorie value
Protein	4 calories/gram
Carbohydrate	4 calories/gram
Fat	9 calories/gram
Alcohol	7 calories/gram
Fiber	1.5-2 calories/gram *

* Note that contrary to popular/past belief, the human body does derive a small amount of calories from fiber. Unless fiber intakes are massive, this simply isn't worth worrying about and I'm going to ignore it from here on out. I'm just including it for completeness.

Step 2: Set protein intake

After calories have been set, I feel that a proper protein intake is the single most important aspect of any diet. This includes fat loss diets, muscle gain diets and maintenance diets. Frankly, no matter what everything else looks like, if protein intake isn't appropriate for the situation, the results will be suboptimal. So before we hassle with carbs or fats, we have to deal with protein.

As I mentioned a chapter or two back, keeping protein higher is turning out to have benefits in terms of weight maintenance in addition to its other benefits and at least one recent study has shown that higher protein intakes after the diet is over help to maintain weight loss. At the very least, it slows weight gain and what weight is regained tends to be LBM. So everybody is going to keep protein intake high.

To simplify things a bit, I'm going to ignore dieting categories here and just focus on activity levels in terms of setting protein intake at maintenance, that will determine how much protein you should be eating at maintenance. In table 3, you'll see suggested protein intakes in grams per pound of lean body mass relative to your activity level

Table 3: Protein recommendations based on activity levels

Activity level	Protein intake (g/lb)
No activity	0.75
Aerobics only	1.0
Weights *	1.5

Includes folks lifting weights and doing aerobics. For more discussion of the debate over protein requirements for athletes, I'd recommend my new book <u>The Protein Book</u>. Please note that recommendations in that book are based on bodyweight and not LBM for reasons discussed in detail in that book.

_____ * _____ = _____
Pound LBM Protein recommendation Grams protein/day

Ok, second annoying math step, you need to multiply your current lean body mass (LBM, not total weight) in pounds by the above value to determine your daily protein intake in grams.

Next annoying math step, multiply total grams of protein by 4 (representing 4 calories per gram) to get your total calories from protein.

_____ * 4 = _____
Grams protein   Calories from protein

Step 3: Set carbohydrate intake

Ok, figuring out how to set up this part of the diet is probably what gave me the biggest headache of this chapter so I'm going to tell you what the problem is (if I must suffer, you must suffer as well). First and foremost, I don't like diets based on percentages because they have literally no relevance to real human physiology. Telling someone to eat 50% of carbs is meaningless except within the context of total calories so such a recommendation is equally meaningless: 50% could be far too high, far too low, or just right depending on the caloric intake of the individual. Rather, nutrient intakes relative to human needs are better expressed in grams per pound, which is what I did with protein previously and above.

The problem is that, within the context of maintenance, giving an across the board g/lb recommendation won't work because I can't predict the body weight of my readers. As well, any carbohydrate recommendation I'd give has to be related to both activity, and insulin resistance, along with a few other variables I'd normally take into account. Trying to get that across simplistically still has me stumped so I'm taking a slightly different approach.

One main factor involved in my decision (and my problem) is that I want people consuming at least 100 grams of carbohydrate per day at maintenance. This is especially true for folks who are just doing a 2 week diet break between periods of dieting and is just another reason that a set g/lb recommendation wouldn't have worked.

There are a number of reasons I'm picking 100 g/day as the bottom end minimum. I already mentioned that at least this many carbs is needed to upregulate thyroid hormone which helps get metabolic rate up and running again. As well, since leptin appears to be sensitive to carbohydrate intake (along with total calories), raising carbs will help raise leptin further helping to fix metabolic rate. This is especially important for people taking a 2 week diet break but also for people looking at long-term maintenance. Additionally, allowing more carbs in the diet allows for more food freedom (while keeping things controlled) which tends to enhance long-term adherence.

Finally, 100 g/day will just avoid ketosis, at least in inactive people. Now, this isn't to say that I think being in ketosis is necessarily bad or dangerous but we simply don't know the extended long-term effect of ketosis. Keeping carbs high enough to just avoid ketosis avoids the problem entirely without putting people for whom carb intake can be a problem right back in the same boat that they were in.

Even then, 100 g/day is generally tolerated by even extremely insulin resistant individuals (though they may need to keep their carb intake limited to vegetables and fruits, no starches). Finally, avoiding ketosis will keep any of your 'well meaning' friends or nutrition experts from bitching at you about how unhealthy ketosis is. Your breath and pee won't smell funny anymore either.

So, what I am going to recommend is that everyone start with a baseline carbohydrate intake of 100 grams/day. That's 100 grams regardless of body weight, activity, or anything else. You may end up at a higher carbohydrate intake because of other factors, but you won't ever go lower.

Ok, the next thing is to add an additional amount of carbs by using one of the multipliers below (which are based on the same activity categories as step one). So if you're sedentary, your multiplier is zero, if you're lightly active, use 0.5, moderately active, 1, etc. What you're going to do is multiply your current lean body mass in pounds by that multiplier factor and then add that number to the 100 grams baseline

So let's say you have a LBM of 150 pounds and have an activity level of lightly active. You'd use a multiplier of 0.5 and multiply that by 150 lbs. to get 75 grams of carbs. You'd add that to the 100 gram/day baseline for a total carbohydrate intake of 175 grams per day. Or say you have 120 pounds of LBM but are extremely active. You'd multiply 120 pounds by 1.5 to get 180 grams and you'd add that to the baseline value of 100 grams for a total of 280 grams of carbohydrate per day. Clearly anyone who is in the sedentary activity level regardless of LBM will be eating only the baseline 100 grams per day of carbs. Recommendations appear in table 4 below.

Table 4: Carbohydrate recommendations based on activity levels

Description	Body weight multiplier (grams)
Sedentary	0
Lightly active	0.5
Moderately active	1
Very active	1.25
Extremely active	1.5

Ok, next annoying math step

_____ * _____ = _____ + 100 g = _____
LBM in pounds Multiplier Grams carbs   Total daily carbs

As well, just as you did for protein, you're now going to multiply the total grams of carbs by 4 (for 4 calories per gram) to get the total number of carbohydrate calories you'll be eating each day.

_____ * 4 = _____
Grams of carbs   Calories from carbs

Step 4: Set fat intake

I promise, you're almost done. The last calculation is to determine daily fat intake by subtracting the number of calories you're getting from protein and carbs from your daily total. Basically, fat intake is simply used as a caloric buffer to make up the rest of your daily calories. So first you need to determine how many calories from you'll be eating by subtracting the number of calories from protein and carbs from your daily total.

_____ - _____ - _____ = _____
Total daily calories   Calories from protein   Calories from carbs   Calories from fat

Now, you will *divide* the total number of fat calories by 9 (representing 9 calories per gram) to get grams of fat per day.

_____ / 9 = _____
Calories from fat   Grams of fat

A note on fiber

I suppose I should mention fiber for completeness. As discussed in the previous 2 chapters, maintaining a high fiber intake (by eating vegetables, fruits and even the higher fiber grains) should be an important part of any diet, including a maintenance diet. Again, since I can't know what diet you're using in applying the information in this booklet, I can only say that I hope it's set up intelligently enough to include lots of vegetables. If it's not, you may want to seriously consider something else. In any event, you should make sure and get plenty of high fiber vegetables in your diet.

Step 5: Putting it all together

Ok, step 5 is simply to gather all of the values from above for easy reference. So take your protein grams from step 2, carb grams from step 3 and fat grams from step 4 and write them below. That's your maintenance diet to be consumed on a daily basis.

Grams protein per day (from Step 2): _____

Grams carbs per day (from Step 3): _____

Grams fat per day (from Step 4): _____

These values would more or less be divided up across however many meals you're choosing to eat (see Chapter 13 for some comments on meal frequency and snacking). Bodybuilders and athletes would typically try to divide those nutrients relatively evenly across their 5-6 (or more) meals but this may not be realistic for everyone. As discussed in Chapter 13, three larger meals with one or more snacks throughout the day may be more attainable for people who can't dedicate their lives to training and eating.

However, and I want to make this point as clearly as possible (this is why I suggested everyone read the previous 2 chapters), any meal or snack should ideally still contain some amount of all the nutrients (and ideally some fiber though this can be a problem). Basically, you should follow the same basic guidelines as described in the past 2 chapters, the only real difference is that you're now keeping more accurate track of your food intake.

In general, I find it best if people pick their protein source first. The reason is that proteins typically either contain some fat (most meats) or carbohydrates (dairy and such). Meaning that you have to figure those values into the overall meal calculation. As a general rule of thumb, most protein sources contain about 7-8 grams of protein per ounce. So 3-4 ounces of most meats will contain 21-30 grams of protein or so. That amount of protein is about the amount that will fit in a cupped palm (or about the size of a deck of cards). Most restaurant portions, for comparison, are typically 2-3 times that amount, 8 oz or more.

Next, ensure your vegetable intake. Think salad, or veggies in that morning omelette, or on your sandwich or whatever. Even rigid calorie counter don't need to worry too much about measuring this, you'd have to eat a metric ton for it to add many calories. The only exceptions, again, are the starchy vegetables carrots, peas and corn which can add a lot of carbohydrate calories to a meal. The bigger issue with salads is usually dressing, as most contain a lot of sugar and fat. The common dieting approach is to get the dressing on the side (and try to pick either a low-cal or low fat version) and dip your food. You'll end up using a lot less of it than if you just try to bury your salad in it.

Fruit would be next and would be applied to your total carbohydrate intake. An average piece of fruit (think apple or banana) is about 20-25 grams of carbs or so. With fruits like grapes or raisins, you'll have to look it up and track it yourself. As mentioned in the last chapter, I think dried fruit is a poor choice, a very small volume can contribute a ton of calories. Fruit juice, as stated, is a horrid choice as far as I'm concerned: it's a glass of concentrated sugar water without any of the fiber or bulk that makes whole fruits such a good food choice.

Next, assuming you have any carbohydrate grams left, you can add a starch if you want. If you're really intolerant to them for some reason, a second piece of fruit can work instead. Starches and whole grains can add a surprising number of carbohydrate calories (especially rice, pasta and the new monster bagels) so read the labels, get out the measuring spoons and figure it out. To give you a few ideas, a typical slice of bread has about 15 grams of carbs, a glass of milk 12, a small baked potato about 25 grams.

Finally, if you haven't used it up with the other foods, you can add your dietary fat. Note again that the foods you've already chosen, even if technically no-fat will have a little bit. If you choose a fattier cut of meat or low-fat or 2% dairy, you've already gotten some as well. But whatever you have left can then be added. Oil and vinegar salad dressings work well and controlled amounts of other fats (think mayo, peanut butter) are acceptable.

As mentioned last chapter, it would be ideal to focus on monounsaturated fats for most of your additional fat intake. You'll get sufficient saturated fats unless you really go out of your way to choose nothing but nonfat meats and dairy and you should still be covering your essential fatty acid requirements from either fish oil capsules or a tablespoon or more of flax oil per day.

What I personally have found works best is this: take the time to sit down and come up with what are essentially modular meals. That is, pick a protein, pick your veggies, add your carbs (fruit/starches), then your fat. Work them out so that they conform to your meal or snack goals. Most people tend to eat more or less the same day in day out, especially if you're looking at the breakfast or lunch meals (dinner tends to be the most variable).

If you have to eat out a lot, figuring out what places allow you to meet your nutritional requirements most easily may be a good thing to do; most places have calorie counts for their foods. For smaller snacks, either work out some mini-meals or find pre-made food bars which meet your requirements for each nutrient.

Although this can be an initial hassle, you'll eventually reach a point where you can just sort of rotate meals as they will be more or less interchangeable. After some time measuring everything, you'll also have a pretty good idea of how to eyeball your foods and get within shooting distance.

Oh yeah, just as with the non-counting approach to maintenance, I still suggest 1 or 2 free meals per week, even if you're counting. Hell, just go read the past chapter, everything I said there applies, you're just counting things now.

Making adjustments

As I mentioned at the first of the chapter, the values I gave for nutrient recommendations are nothing but estimates upon estimates and should not be taken as anything more than that. At the end of the day, real world changes in your body composition, weight or fat (again this necessitates regular monitoring) should be your ultimate goal. If your weight is slowly climbing, you need to cut something back or increase your activity.

In general, I'd say cut back your carbohydrate (starches and grains, fruits if you have to) intake a bit. Cutting back fat slightly is another option although very low fat diets tend to backfire, as I've mentioned, leaving people hungrier at the end of the day. Under no circumstances do I think you should cut your protein intake. Or your vegetables.

If you're still in a situation where your weight is moving down slowly, well, you have a couple of options. If further weight loss is your goal, you can just run with it. If you are more interested in weight stability for the time being, increase your food intake slightly. Carbohydrates or fats would be the best bet here.

In neither case should huge changes be necessary or made. If your weight is gradually creeping up, try cutting 100-200 calories out of your diet. That would mean either a 25-50 gram reduction in carbohydrates or about a 10-20 gram reduction in fat. Same for weight loss but in reverse, add a couple of hundred calories per day until weight stabilizes. This is discussed in more detail in the final chapter.

96

Moving Back Into Dieting

Ok, one more chapter and this book is done. The previous three chapters dealt with how to move to maintenance using one of two different approaches: a non-calculating method (Chapter 13 and 14) and a pain in the ass method where you calculate your nutrient requirements and measure your food (Chapter 15). The information presented in those chapters applies for the full diet break, as well as when dieters finally decide to end their diet and move to maintenance.

This chapter is sort of a snapshot view of what I think constitutes a good fat loss diet, in terms of how it should be set up and how it should be adjusted based on real world fat loss. One of these days, when I finally get my act together, I'm going to take this information, along with a host of other stuff I've written and put together my be-all, end-all guidebook to dieting. For the time being you're stuck with the abbreviated version.

What is a realistic expectation from a diet?

So how quickly can you really lose weight or fat? With the exception of extreme approaches like the one described in my last booklet, a 1-2 pound week true fat loss is about all that can realistically be expected with a more moderate or traditional type of calorically restricted diet. Extremely large or fatter individuals will often lose somewhat more (maybe 3-4 pounds) but lighter individuals should be more than happy with a consistent weekly fat loss of 1-2 pounds.

Now, this may seem pretty pathetic compared to a lot of the claims that are made for so many diets, promises of 5-10 pounds per week are often made. And, well, that's true under certain conditions for very short periods of time. Usually it's when you take a very fat individual and put them on an extremely low-carbohydrate diet. For the first couple of weeks, they drop a ton of water weight and that can easily add up to 5-10 pounds or more weight loss in a very short period of time. Then, invariably, total weekly weight and/or fat loss slows way down to about the ranges I gave above. Again, lighter or leaner individuals can be lucky to get 1-1.5 pounds of true fat loss per week but I'm getting ahead of myself.

Now, if you are simply using the strategies in this booklet in conjunction with a diet that you are already on, you can probably safely ignore what I'm going to write. Just finish your full diet break and then move back into dieting like you were before. You should lose fat as effectively as you were, if not more so.

Of course, I'm assuming here that the diet you were following to begin with was producing results as desired. If not, perhaps you want a bit more in the way of guidelines for moving back into a traditional type of fat loss diet. So I'm going to go into a bit more detail about how I think a proper fat loss diet should be set up, mainly in terms of setting up caloric deficits.

The three primary requirements of any fat loss diet

Back on page 25, I made some comments about a few of the requirements that I think any good fat loss diet should meet and I want to review them here. The first one, and the one that this chapter is mainly going to deal with, is that a diet must cause an imbalance between calorie intake and calorie burning. That fundamental law of thermodynamics, that so many diet books tell you doesn't apply to humans (yet somehow applies to everything else in the universe) is the fundamental aspect of a diet in my opinion. Short of manipulating water balance, if a diet doesn't cause an imbalance between intake and output, very little (if anything) will happen.

A second aspect is that a good fat loss diet must provide sufficient protein. A lot of mainstream diets are protein deficient as far as I'm concerned and this does nothing to improve their success rate. We've known for nearly three decades that protein requirements go up as calories go down and recent studies are finding that diets with higher protein (for example 25% of total calories versus 12% of total calories) are more effective in a lot of ways. Frankly, if you followed my recommendations for protein intake from the previous chapters and simply maintain that as you move back into dieting, you should be fine.

For dieting purposes, bodybuilders and athletes have long used a value of 1 gram of protein per pound of lean body mass (or higher in some situations) and while that might be overkill for someone not involved in heavy training, I'd rather see people get slightly too much protein than too little. As long as you make sure to get a reasonable amount of protein at every meal (3 oz or 21-24 grams as a bare minimum), you should be fine. I think you'll find that your hunger/appetite is better controlled and your diet works better than with a lower protein intake.

A final requirement for a proper fat loss diet is that it should provide some essential fatty acids, primarily the w-3 fatty acids. Once again, fish oil capsules are my preferred option but flax oil is another possibility. If you applied my recommendations from the past chapters, this should be a non-issue as well. I suppose mandating a high fiber intake from vegetables should be on that list, it's nearly impossible to go wrong eating lots of vegetables unless you insist on burying them in high-fat cheeses or dressings.

Beyond that, the setup of a fat loss diet depends on a host of factors including activity, genetics, food preferences, etc. It's stuff that I sort of simplified in the last chapter but are somewhat complicated to get across in detail in a book format. I'll get it done eventually, but not in this project.

In any event, I'm going to focus primarily on the issue of calorie balance and making adjustments to them based on real-world fat loss.

The typical approach to calorie restriction

In a previous chapter, I mentioned the diets that take an 'Eat as much as you want as long as you do X' where 'X' may be 'don't eat carbs', 'reduce fat', or 'only mix and match certain types of foods'. As far as I'm concerned, they all work by picking an eating strategy that tends to make people eat less automatically. Frankly, when such diets work, as long as they meet protein and fatty acid requirements, I have no beef with them. Any diet that gets you to eat less without having to obsess about it too much is a good thing in my book. My problem, as mentioned previously, is that they often don't work out as planned. Humans can usually find really amusing ways to eat more than they think and such diets end up failing as often as not.

There are also the diets that steadfastly tell you that you don't have to count or restrict calories and then set the diet up so that you invariably do so anyhow. They'll hide the caloric restriction in the diet setup itself but when you actually sit down and work out your caloric intake, it's always way below maintenance.

Ignoring those two broad categories of diet are the ones that actually do give specific calorie intake recommendations. Those are the ones I want to discuss in a bit more detail. Typically, diets take one of two approaches to setting daily calories.

A standard approach to a weight loss diet would be to recommend some fixed calorie level to everyone, although usually men and women are given different recommendations (i.e. 1200 and 1500-1800 cal/day for men and women respectively). I consider this approach rather ludicrous. For those of you who read the last chapter, it should be clear that maintenance calorie requirements depends on both activity level and body weight. To suggest that all men, regardless of weight and activity should eat the same number of calories per day is either ignorant or just plain lazy. Perhaps a bit of both.

Another typical approach would be to recommend that everyone reduce their daily caloric intake by anywhere from 500-1000 calories per day, depending on whether they want a 1 or 2 pound weight loss per week. As the math and logic go, since one pound of fat contains 3,500 calories, if you eat 500 calories/day less, you will lose one pound of fat per week; 1000 calories per day less and you will lose two. It never works out that perfectly (people never seem to lose exactly the predicted amount of fat per week that the numbers indicate) for reasons unimportant to this booklet but I don't want to get into that.

Rather I want to point out the problem with giving an absolute caloric reduction for everyone: the same absolute caloric reduction has staggeringly different effects on total daily caloric intake. Again, the issue has to do with body weight, activity and maintenance calorie intakes. If a light female, who may have a maintenance requirement of about 1700 calories/day reduces her food intake by 500 calories, she's at 1200. If she reduces her total food intake by 1000, she's at 700 cal/day. This is not very much food. By the same token, a large male with a maintenance intake of 3500 calories is still at a rather hefty 3000 cal/day with a 500 cal/day reduction, and 2500 cal/day if he reduces 1000 calories. Basically, a flat daily caloric reduction doesn't take into account the variance in estimated intake: lighter individuals end up taking a much larger drop (as a percentage of their maintenance), and end up at a much lower absolute intake level than heavier individuals.

I don't like either of the above methods. The first is simply silly, no single caloric recommendation can possibly apply across the board. Even if you split it up into male and female recommendations, it's still absurd to think that all females should eat the same number of calories regardless of weight or activity. The second is equally problematic as the same absolute caloric reduction tends to have drastically different effects on food intake depending on the person's current maintenance needs.

My preferred method

My preferred method, as I originally described in my book The Ketogenic Diet, then is to simply reduce food intake relative to your current daily maintenance level. This means that any reductions are made relative to what you actually need to eat (or are currently eating, assuming your weight is stable). So the person eating only 1700 calories/day has a smaller food reduction than someone eating 3000 calories/day. Since I've described two different approaches for moving to maintenance, I have to make comments for each.

For folks using the non-measurement method described in Chapters 13 and 14, that would basically mean just reducing their food intake slightly from what they are eating now. My primary recommendation would be to cut back on concentrated starches first (which tend to contribute the most calories without doing a great job of filling people up), fat intake can be reduced slightly (I wouldn't go less than one half tablespoon or 7 grams of fat per meal, though) or some of the fruit can be dropped out. At no point should protein or vegetable intake be reduced. Making these types of small changes will reduce daily caloric intake slightly and get fat loss moving.

That small reduction in food intake would be maintained for several weeks and then the person would look at their weight/fat loss. As above, short of extreme approaches, a realistic weekly fat loss is usually 1-2 pounds. Lighter women may be lucky to get 1 pound/week but heavier/fatter individuals can often get more. But based on real world changes, further reductions could be made based on what is actually happening. So if you're losing less than one pound per week on average, you can reduce your food intake (or increase activity) slightly more until you hit the sweet spot. See the chart below for more comments on this.

If someone were calculating nutrients as per the last chapter, I'd have them reduce their food intake by 10-20% per day from what they are eating at maintenance. So if they had a maintenance level of 3000 cal/day based on activity and body weight, they'd reduce by 300-600 calories/day. If they had a maintenance of 1700 cal/day, they'd reduce by 170-340 calories/day. Which means that, if they are using the method from the last chapter, they have to go recalculate their carb and fat intakes based on that change to their daily caloric intake.

As always, protein intake stays the same, with the adjustment coming to carbohydrate and fat intake. As above, it may simply be easiest for dieters to reduce their concentrated carbohydrate (starch) intakes to achieve the calorie reduction. Or use some mix of carbohydrate and fat reduction.

After adjusting their food intake, they'd stay at that level for 2-3 weeks and track changes in body composition. Based on real world changes, they'd make adjustments according to the scheme below.

Average weekly fat loss	Change to caloric intake
Less than 1 lb/week	Reduce calories by 10%
1-1.5 lb/week	No change
2+ pounds/week:	
Category 1 dieters involved in heavy training	
No performance loss	No change
Performance loss	Increase calories by 10%
Category 2 and 3 dieters	No change

The first two situations should be fairly clear to most people. If you're losing less than one pound per week on average, and you're not an extremely light female, you need to cut calories further, another 10% reduction would be appropriate. Then maintain that for 2-3 weeks and re-measure.

Anybody who is losing a consistent 1-1.5 pounds per week is basically in the sweet spot, they shouldn't change a thing. If they are in dieting Category 2 or 3, they can consider a further 10% calorie reduction to see if they can achieve a slightly higher weekly fat loss. Frankly, anyone achieving 1-1.5 pounds/week on a consistent basis is doing really well.

The most complicated situation, as the chart above indicates is whether or not a loss of greater than 2 pounds per week (again, this is under moderate dieting conditions) is need for alarm. Basically, it depends on the circumstances.

A Category 2 or 3 dieter may have no problem losing that much weight weekly and probably shouldn't adjust calories. The real issue is for Category 1 dieters, especially if they are involved in high intensity activity, a loss that great might signal muscle/LBM loss. Category 1 dieters involved in heavy training should use their performance or strength as the deciding factor. If they are losing 2 lbs./week and NOT losing strength or seeing a decrement in performance, they are probably ok. But they should be very alert to the possibility of overtraining, performance loss, and muscle loss. If strength in the gym or athletic performance is showing a large drop, Category 1 dieters should increase calories by 10%.

A couple of random comments about the above chart

I should mention that, rather than reducing caloric intake by 10%, it is also possible to increase activity (via exercise) instead. So let's assume that someone is currently eating 2000 calories/day and losing less than one pound per week. If, for some reason, they didn't want to decrease their calories (by 10% or 200 calories), they could increase their activity level to burn an additional 200 calories instead. By the same token, if someone were losing too quickly, rather than increase their food intake by 10%, they could reduce the amount of activity they were doing.

I bring this up because dieters often run into situations where further reductions in calories are simply unrealistic; this is especially true when caloric intakes get very low. In those situations, adding activity may be the only way to create a suitable deficit. This is especially true for women and lighter men; their daily caloric requirements are so low to begin with that there is a very real limit to how far food intake can be reduced. They are probably better off increasing activity.

I should also mention that it is exceedingly rare for fat loss to occur in a linear or nonstop fashion. Rather, it's not uncommon for stalls of several weeks to occur followed by major drops in scale weight and changes in appearance. Empirically, these drops often occur after performing a structured refeed. My guess is that it has to do with screwy water balance on a diet but I can't really support that with any hard data. I've simply seen it occur enough times to know that it happens.

I bring this up for the following reason: let's say that you've made an alteration to your food intake and stayed there for 2-3 weeks. Now it looks like nothing is happening. By the above chart, you need to reduce food intake (or increase activity), right? Well, maybe. It may very well be that, given another week (or by incorporating a structured refeed), things will start moving. I can't give any really super accurate guidelines for what you should do; simply be aware that an apparent zero change over a few weeks may suddenly become 'apparent' rather rapidly. Again, I can't explain why it works this way, only that it does.

Another method for setting calories

I should probably mention another popular method of setting daily calories, one that I also described in my first book (not that I was writing about anything very new). Remember from the last chapter that the average person will typically have a daily maintenance caloric requirement of 14-16 calories per pound or so. Well, many authors simply take a 20% reduction in calories from that starting point which puts most people in about the

11-12 calorie/pound level. More often, a range of 10-12 calories/pound for dieting is used; people with low activity levels should use 10 calories/pound, people with medium activity levels should use 11 and people with high activity levels should use 12 calories/pound.

Frankly, this isn't a bad way to set starting calorie levels on a diet, but they often still need to be adjusted. I've seen people, usually with very low activity levels (and often with a general resistance towards fat loss) who have to reduce calories to 8 calories/pound to achieve reasonable levels of fat loss. Some metabolically hapless individuals may have to go to 8 calories per pound and increase activity levels quite a bit to get fat loss moving.

If you choose to use this method, simply go back into the last chapter (or use whatever diet you're currently using) and use a value of 10-12 calories per pound to determine your starting caloric intake. Then stay there for several weeks as above, noting real world weight/fat loss. Then make adjustments as the above chart suggests.

Appendix 1: BMI and Body fat estimation charts

As discussed in the main text of this book, BMI can be used to roughly estimate body fat percentage and readers can use Table 1, 2 and 3 (or the online calculator) to first estimate BMI (Table 1 and 2) and then estimate body fat percentage (Table 3). I want to make it abundantly clear again that active individuals should not and can not use this method to estimate body fat percentage, they must find another method. Dieters shorter than 5'7" should use Table 1 while those 5'8" and above should use Table 2 on the next page.

Table 1: BMI Chart Part 1 (Short-folks)

Feet		4'10	4'11	5'0	5'1	5'2	5'3	5'4	5'5	5'6	5'7
Meters		1.47	1.5	1.52	1.55	1.57	1.60	1.63	1.65	1.68	1.70
Lb	Kg										
100	45	21	20	20	19	18	18	17	17	16	16
110	50	23	22	22	21	20	20	19	18	18	17
120	55	25	24	23	23	22	21	21	20	19	19
130	60	27	26	25	25	24	23	22	22	21	20
140	64	29	28	27	26	26	25	24	23	23	22
150	68	31	30	29	28	28	27	26	25	24	24
160	73	33	32	31	30	29	28	28	27	26	25
170	77	36	34	33	32	31	30	29	28	28	27
180	82	38	36	35	34	33	32	31	30	29	28
190	86	40	38	37	36	35	34	33	32	31	30
200	91	42	40	39	38	37	35	34	33	32	31
210	95	44	43	41	40	39	37	36	35	34	33
220	100	46	45	43	42	40	39	38	37	36	35
230	105	48	47	45	44	42	41	40	39	37	36
240	109	50	49	47	45	44	43	41	40	39	38
250	114	53	51	49	47	46	45	43	42	41	39
260	118	54	53	51	49	48	46	45	43	42	41
270	123	57	55	53	51	50	48	47	45	44	42
280	127	59	57	55	53	51	50	48	47	45	44
290	132	61	59	57	55	53	52	50	48	47	46
300	136	63	61	59	57	55	53	51	50	48	47
310	141	65	63	61	59	57	55	53	52	50	49
320	145	67	65	62	60	58	57	55	53	52	50
330	150	69	67	65	62	60	59	57	55	53	52
340	155	71	69	67	65	63	61	59	57	55	54
350	159	73	71	68	66	64	62	60	58	57	55
360	164	76	73	71	68	66	64	62	60	58	57
370	168	77	75	72	70	68	66	64	62	60	58
380	173	80	77	75	72	70	68	66	64	62	60
390	177	82	79	76	74	71	69	67	65	63	61
400	182	84	81	78	76	73	71	69	67	65	63

Table 2: BMI Chart Part 2 (Tall folks)

Feet		5'8	5'9	5'10	5'11	6'0	6'1	6'2	6'3	6'4
Meters		1.73	1.75	1.78	1.80	1.83	1.85	1.88	1.91	1.93
Lb	Kg									
100	45	15	15	14	14	14	13	13	13	12
110	50	17	16	16	15	15	15	14	14	13
120	55	18	18	17	17	16	16	15	15	15
130	60	20	19	19	18	18	17	17	16	16
140	64	21	21	20	20	19	18	18	18	17
150	68	23	22	22	21	20	20	19	19	18
160	73	24	24	23	22	22	21	21	20	20
170	77	26	25	24	24	23	22	22	21	21
180	82	27	27	26	25	24	24	23	23	22
190	86	29	28	27	27	26	25	24	24	23
200	91	30	30	29	28	27	26	26	25	24
210	95	32	31	30	29	29	28	27	26	26
220	100	34	33	32	31	30	29	28	28	27
230	105	35	34	33	32	31	31	30	29	28
240	109	37	35	34	34	33	32	31	30	29
250	114	38	37	36	35	34	33	32	31	31
260	118	40	38	37	36	35	34	33	33	32
270	123	41	40	39	38	37	36	35	34	33
280	127	43	41	40	39	38	37	36	35	34
290	132	44	43	42	41	39	38	37	36	35
300	136	46	44	43	42	41	40	38	37	36
310	141	47	46	45	43	42	41	40	39	38
320	145	49	47	46	45	43	42	41	40	39
330	150	50	49	47	46	45	44	42	41	40
340	155	52	50	49	48	46	45	44	43	42
350	159	53	52	50	49	48	46	45	44	43
360	164	55	53	52	50	49	48	46	45	44
370	168	56	55	53	52	50	49	48	46	45
380	173	58	57	55	54	52	51	49	48	47
390	177	59	58	56	54	53	51	50	49	47
400	182	61	59	58	56	54	53	52	50	49

To determine BMI, locate your height on the top row (the top value is height in feet and inches, the bottom is meters) and then cross-reference it with weight on the left hand column (left most column is weight in pounds, right column is weight in kilograms).

So an individual who is 5'0" (1.52 meters) tall and 150 pounds (68 kilograms) will have a BMI of 28. If your weight falls in between two values, simply take the halfway value of the two. So a 5'2" (1.57 meter) individual weighing 165 pounds (~75 kg) would estimate their BMI halfway between the 160 and 170 lb values of 26 and 28 to get a BMI of 27.

Once you have your BMI, use table 2 to get a rough estimate of your body fat percentage. Once again please note that this is only an estimate and that active and/or athletic individuals cannot use this method, as it will drastically misestimate them. It is for inactive people only.

Table 2: BMI and Body fat percentage

BMI	Female BF%	Male BF%	BMI	Female BF%	Male BF%
13	13.5	You are dead	27	34.5	21.5
14	15	You are dead	28	36	23
15	16.5	You are dead	29	37.5	24.5
16	18	5	30	39	26
17	19.5	6.5	31	40.5	27.5
18.5	21	8	32	42	29
19	22.5	9.5	33	43.5	30.5
20	24	11	34	45	32
21	25.5	12.5	35	46.5	33.5
22	27	14	36	48	35
23	28.5	15.5	37	49.5	36.5
24	30	17	38	51	38
25	31.5	18.5	39	52.5	39.5
26	33	20	40	54	41

Note: If your BMI is over 40, add 1.5% body fat for each BMI point.

My Other Books

Depending on what your typical reading materials are, you may or may not be familiar with my other books (I mean beyond my endless mentioning of them in the text of this booklet) so I thought I'd bring them to your attention in case you are at all interested in what else I have written.   All of them can be ordered through my website at http://www.bodyrecomposition.com

The Protein Book: A Complete Guide for the Athlete and Coach (Published 2007)

Similar to my first book on the ketogenic diet, The Protein Book is a comprehensive look at the topic of dietary protein for athletes. Every topic from basic protein metabolism, protein requirements, nutrient timing around training and supplements is discussed. As well, each whole food protein and protein powder is examine in terms of its pros and cons for athletes. Of course, how to put all of the information together for different kinds of athletes (strength/power, endurance, physique) is included. The book is over 200 pages and includes over 500 scientific references.

The Rapid Fat Loss Handbook (Published 2005)

The Rapid Fat Loss handbook describes a low-carbohydrate, low-calorie crash diet capable of causing total weight losses of 10-20 pounds and actual fat losses of 4-7 pounds in only two weeks. How to set up the diet, how optimally to train, in addition to many chapters dealing with coming off the diet present an integrated system of training and nutrition for the most rapid fat losses possible.

The Ultimate Diet 2.0 (Published 2004)

I must have mentioned my UD2 a dozen or more times in the text of this booklet. The UD2 is an updating of the original Ultimate Diet that was written nearly 20 years ago. It is a diet for hardcore dieters who are already very lean (12-15% body fat or lower for men) and who want to get even leaner without losing any muscle.

The Ketogenic Diet: A Complete Guide for the Dieter and Practitioner (Published 1998).

This was my first project and it's a monster. It's 325 pages of information dense text with over 600 scientific references. To say that it is the be-all, end-all guidebook for low-carbohydrate/ketogenic diets is an understatement. There's really no other book in its category. I should note that it is written in a very different style than this booklet or my others; it's somewhat dry and very technical. It covers nutritional and exercise physiology and gives recommendations for three different types of low-carbohydrate diets, as well as sample exercise programs from beginner to advanced. It is really for the hardcore low-carbohydrate dieter who truly wants to know everything that is going on in their body when they are in ketosis.

Bromocriptine: An Old Drug with a New Use (Published 2002)

My second booklet is sort of incorrectly named. Ostensibly it's about a drug called Bromocriptine (which has been used for the treatment of Parkinson's disease for about 30 years) but it really delves into the details of body weight regulation in some detail. I don't even mention the titular drug until about Chapter 6, the first 5 chapters are all about body weight regulation. This booklet is fully referenced and written in a more conversational and readable style than my first. It is available only as an e-book.

110